Be Fit For Life:
A Guide To Successful Aging

A Wellness, Weight Management,
and Fitness Program You Can Live With

Be Fit For Life:
A Guide To Successful Aging

A Wellness, Weight Management,
and Fitness Program You Can Live With

Steven R Gambert, MD, AGSF, MACP
University of Maryland School of Medicine and
Johns Hopkins University School of Medicine, USA

Professor of Medicine and Associate Chairman
Clinical Director,
Division of Gerontology and Geriatric Medicine
Department of Medicine
University of Maryland School of Medicine

Director of Geriatric Medicine
University of Maryland Medical Center and
R Adams Cowley Shock Trauma Center

Professor of Medicine
Division of Gerontology and Geriatric Medicine
Department of Medicine
Johns Hopkins University School of Medicine

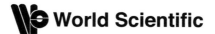

NEW JERSEY · LONDON · SINGAPORE · BEIJING · SHANGHAI · HONG KONG · TAIPEI · CHENNAI

Published by

World Scientific Publishing Co. Pte. Ltd.

5 Toh Tuck Link, Singapore 596224

USA office: 27 Warren Street, Suite 401-402, Hackensack, NJ 07601

UK office: 57 Shelton Street, Covent Garden, London WC2H 9HE

British Library Cataloguing-in-Publication Data
A catalogue record for this book is available from the British Library.

BE FIT FOR LIFE: A GUIDE TO SUCCESSFUL AGING
A Wellness, Weight Management, and Fitness Program You Can Live With

ISBN-13 978-981-4273-09-1 (pbk)
ISBN-10 981-4273-09-0 (pbk)

Typeset by Stallion Press
Email: enquiries@stallionpress.com

Printed in Singapore.

Dedication

This book is dedicated to my family who moment by moment provide me with the inspiration to do my very best to Age Successfully. I am particularly indebted to my wife, Gry, and my daughter, Iselin, for their valuable suggestions to me while writing this book. Each of them has provided me with invaluable wisdom over the years and given me many ideas for exploration as well as excellent practical advice. My son, Christopher, his wife Kjersti, and my grandson, Storm have also taught me much about appreciating the many pleasures life has to offer and how best to "recalibrate" when necessary in order to achieve a lifetime of Successful Aging.

Contents

1

Introduction

"Man Fools himself. He prays for a long life, and he fears an old age."

— Chinese proverb

Do you want to live to blow out 100 candles on your birthday cake? Would you like those extra years to be filled with productive activity, enjoyment, and meaning? Would you prefer to stay fit and maintain a radiantly youthful appearance throughout your life? You are not alone and the answer is within easy reach!

The search for eternal youth and good health has preoccupied mankind for centuries. Initially, alchemists and explorers searched for some rejuvenating "power", be it an elixer or some natural substance. Although modern times have added some degree of scientific knowledge to the search, the "Fountain of Youth" is still a highly sought after prize.

While it is unlikely that a "magic potion" capable of altering the aging process will ever be found, each of us has within our own power the ability to live longer, healthier, more productive and happy lives. Although we cannot change many factors, such as our genetic makeup, we can certainly control many aspects of our lives. Science has shown that modifications in our lifestyle and environment can lead to the maintenance of good health, prevention of disease, and a high quality of life as our bodies undergo the natural aging process.

Aging occurs throughout life with no clear demarcation between periods of youth, maturity, and senescence. While our birth certificates provide a chronological age for comparison, our physiological or biological age more accurately reflects the way our bodies actually function with some dividing this even further to include a separate and measurable functional age. These forms of aging may or may not run in parallel; our genetic make-up and lifelong exposure to a variety of environmental factors, including diet, exercise, lifestyle, among many other variables, will determine just how "successful" one's individual aging process will actually be. In brief, we have the ability to lead healthier, more active, and rewarding lives — it is up to each of us to make this a reality.

Unfortunately, as we age, many of us neglect ourselves. We may eat less than an ideal diet gaining weight and increasing our risk of developing heart disease, diabetes, high blood pressure, and stroke. Even having healthy bones demands proper diet throughout one's life. A sedentary lifestyle will result in reduced tolerance for everyday activities, weight gain, loss of vital muscle mass and bone strength while increasing one's risk of developing certain diseases including heart disease and diabetes. While stressful situations may not easily be avoided, the way we "deal" with life's stressful situations varies greatly from person to person. Numerous stress reduction techniques can be mastered for a healthier and happier life.

The literature is filled with empty promises, testimonials, and at times, unsafe and unproven techniques and diets. Even some nutritional supplements and "natural" products may not be as safe as one might be led to believe. Not everyone will benefit from the same diet, exercise program, or life changing process. Individualization is key if one is to not only achieve success in reaching one's goals, but also maintain these goals throughout life.

A healthier YOU is within easy reach. Your individualized Prescription for a Healthy Life as outlined in this book can easily be achieved. Simply incorporate the information provided in this book into your everyday life; it has been specifically designed to meet your specific needs, desires, and goals. The information provided in this book is based on scientific evidence and many years of experience. *Be Fit for Life* is designed with YOU in mind!

2

Step One: Preventing an Accelerated Aging Process

A Journey of a Thousand Miles Begins with the First Step …

— Confucius

Aging is a life-long process from which no person can escape, yet no one needs to fear. Regardless of one's sex, race, religion, or place of origin, we all share certain genetically pre-determined changes affecting every cell, organ, and system in the body. Although these changes occur throughout our lives, there is a great deal of individual variability as to how rapidly they occur. While I would be lying if I told you that an inherent aging process can be prevented, we hold the keys in our hands as to just how "successful" our aging process will be. While aging cannot be "prevented", it can be "accelerated", something we want to avoid at all stages in our lives. Foods we eat or fail to eat, environmental factors, diseases, and changes in lifestyle can all cause us to age faster than our biological clocks intended. This does not have to happen to YOU!

The GOOD NEWS is that we are born with a tremendous reserve capability and it is NEVER TOO LATE to take steps that can halt the acceleration of the aging process and improve one's health, happiness, and endurance. In short, we are in control of our own health and bodies — the choice, however, is ours to make and keep.

Many persons unnecessarily enter a downward spiral that depletes their reserves and results in a less than optimal quality of life. While few realize that changes are taking place throughout their lives, every moment our bodies undergo change. We all have the potential to grow and improve or to diminish and fail.

Perhaps one of the most common findings we notice as we age is our changing body habitus. Once we reach our 30's, it becomes increasingly difficult for many of us to maintain the body shape and the same weight that we were accustomed to earlier in our lives. For some of us, our lives have taken us down a path of inactivity and thus a reduced ability to metabolize the calories we eat. For others, poor eating practices may have led to an imbalance between calories taken in and expended with resultant weight gain. With age, however, there are changes in the way we are able to metabolize the calories we ingest even if we do nothing different from our past practices; there is a great deal of variability from person to person. Many of us will need to adjust our diet and increase the amount of exercise we are getting as we age merely to maintain a desirable weight and muscle mass; many persons, however, will need to be on a calorie restricted diet to loose that unwanted weight that has slowly become problematic over the years and if not corrected, potentially life-threatening.

While many years ago it was felt that weight should be constant throughout life and those who were thinner lived longer, Reuben Andres, MD of the National Institute of Aging reported in a landmark study that longevity correlated best with a "U Shaped Curve". This meant that with age, individuals who started out life thin and gained some weight over time actually lived longer. Those who were "too thin" or "overweight", died earlier. Based on this data, the Metropolitan Life Insurance Company adjusted their standard weight tables upward as one aged and expressed the recommended ranges as "Average Weight for Age". Men were still considered to be "average" at a higher weight than women given their greater degree of muscle mass and bone structure at any age. It appears, however, that gaining at least some weight as we age, as long as it is not excessive, provides us with that extra "margin of safety" when we are older. At this time in life, we have less reserve and ability to deal with stressful situations such as infections and illness that may lead us to have a reduced dietary intake and increased metabolism. Too much weight gain as we age, however, increases our risk of developing certain age-prevalent diseases and changes our ability to function optimally. The trick is to get on track for a lifetime of proper diet, exercise, and lifestyle modification in order to have a Successful Aging Process.

Normal Aging is a term that describes what happens to all of us to varying degrees and variable rates throughout our lives. Genetic make-up is perhaps the most important variable as to how successful we will be as we age, though even here, we have within our power the ability to maximize our potential to its fullest! Wrinkling of the skin, graying of the hair, and a decreased ability to increase one's heart rate in response to exercise are just a few changes that occur in all of us as we grow older.

In general, processes that involve only single parameters, such as a nerve conducting an electrical impulse from your shoulder to your fingers, change little if any with increasing age. While scientists can detect differences using sophisticated experimental equipment between such findings in the 30 year old and the 80 year old, for example, differences between the 30 and 40 or 40 and

60 year old are not so obvious and in all cases have little, if any, clinical consequences and no untoward effect on one's daily functioning. Even the 80 year old under normal circumstances who goes to pick up a pot of boiling noodles, for example, can sense the hot sensation and "let go" in sufficient time to not burn themselves or drop the pot. If that same 80 year old had some disease or trauma to the nerves, however, the decline in nerve conduction speed that everyone has as part of the normal aging process might be more advanced than would otherwise be the case; the simple act of touching a hot pot might now result in significant harm due to a delay in response time between receiving the message and being able to respond appropriately.

Processes that involve an integration of several parameters, such as how our kidneys work, are more critically affected by age. These processes decline at an even faster rate, though even here, age-related changes do not have any significant effect in themselves if allowed to progress as nature intended. Using the kidney as an example, the kidney has an approximate drop in function of 0.6% per year after the age of 30. This decline, while significant, has little impact on one's overall health status. It may, however, mandate that there be an adjustment in the dose of a medication that is eliminated through the kidney. As before, diseases or processes that "accelerate" the otherwise "normal" decline in kidney function lead to situations where there may be a need for a change in diet, and may result in clinical findings associated with an inability to excrete toxic wastes such as ammonia. Physicians often over estimate how well the kidneys work in older people because the blood test that is most commonly used to measure kidney function, serum creatinine, is a product of muscle breakdown and our ability to excrete creatinine through the kidneys. Since older persons have a decline in muscle mass with age, they have less creatinine released from muscle to be broken down. Therefore even a "normal" serum creatinine level may not represent normal kidney function. In general, an 80 year old individual with a "normal" serum creatinine level has approximately 40% of the kidney function they had earlier in life.

When one examines processes that demand many body functions to work together in a coordinated manner much like a well-tuned automobile, changes with age become more significant. Two such examples are our ability to run a marathon and survive outside in a blizzard. Even here there are ways of improving our abilities at any age. For example, peak marathon performance tends to occur between our late 20's and early 30's. Nevertheless, there are numerous individuals over the age of 80 who are able to run this distance, though not at the same speed if they had trained for a similar amount of time when they were younger. Older persons die more frequently from hypothermia, or a drop in body temperature below a healthy level. While there are many different reasons for this to occur, studies have demonstrated an approximate 2 degree Fahrenheit difference in the ambient room temperature between when a younger and older person first notes a change in environmental temperature and seeks assistance to stay "warm". The body has two mechanisms to increase core body temperature, shivering and non-shivering thermogenesis. When the older person feels "cold", they start to shiver; since older persons have less muscle mass as compared to those who are younger, this effort is not as effective in raising body temperature. The body also has a series of metabolic processes that attempt to increase body temperature at the cellular level with catecholamines and thyroid hormone playing significant roles. With age, these may not be as effective and medications and illness more common during later life may also impair this effect. Older persons may need to compete with younger individuals for places that provide warmth as well as afford heating fuel to keep their homes at a suitable temperature. Remember, however, that we are continually in a temperature producing mode even to keep our body temperature at the normal 98.6 F (37C) degrees. Since room temperature is usually set between 68 and 72 degrees Fahrenheit, everyday circumstances may result in "hypothermia" if the body does not work appropriately to maintain our needed body temperature.

While age does take a toll, it must not be considered a barrier to doing things one never dreamed were possible. We have the ability to improve our physical state at any point in our lives. The choice, however, is ours to make.

Examples of Normal Age-Related Changes

Central Nervous System

— decline in the number of neurons and the weight of the brain; reduced short-term memory; takes longer to learn new information; slowing of reaction time

Spinal Cord/Peripheral Nerves

— decline in nerve conduction velocity; diminished sensation; decline in the number of fibers in the nerve trunks; decline in reaction time

Cardiovascular System

— reduced cardiac output; valvular sclerosis of the aortic valves; reduced ability to increase heart rate in response to exercise; thickening of arterial intima

Respiratory System

— decline in capacity of lungs; increased residual lung volume; increased anterior-posterior chest diameter; reduced ciliary action

Gastrointestinal System

— reduced number of taste buds; loss of dentition; reduced gastric acid secretion; decreased ability to absorb various nutrients including calcium; reduced motility of large intestine

Genito-urinary System

— loss of nephrons in the kidney; reduced glomerular filtration rate and tubular reabsorption; change in renal threshold for excretion

Musculoskeletal System

— loss of bone density (normal?); reduced cartilage in joints; diminished lean muscle mass

Endocrine/Metabolic System

— reduced basal metabolic rate; reduced glucose tolerance; changes in thyroid hormone economy; menopause; decline in free testosterone; decreased cortisol production; increased anti-diuretic hormone

Reproductive System

men   — delayed penile erection; less frequent orgasm; increased refractory period after sex; decreased sperm motility and altered morphology

women — decreased vaso-congestion; delayed/reduced vaginal lubrication; diminished orgasm; ovarian atrophy.

Skin

— loss of elasticity; atrophy of sweat glands; hair loss

Sensory

Eye: arcus senilis; lenticular opacity; decreased pupillary size; contraction of visual fields; yellowing of the lens

Ears: atrophy of external auditory canal opening; atrophy of cochlear hair cells; decreased high frequency hearing

Taste: reduced number of taste buds; decline in taste sensation

Smell: decline in the sensation of smell

If aging is inevitable and we cannot change our genetics, then what can we do to live longer, happier and healthier lives? One answer lies in taking steps to insure that our aging is NOT accelerated.

3

Step 2: Preventing Disease

Disease is Not an Inevitable Consequence of Growing Old

Many persons confuse changes that result from normal aging with disease. Often older persons and their relatives accept poor health as an inevitable consequence of growing older. This acceptance has been fostered by a lack of understanding of many of the problems of old age as well as a nihilistic attitude by many health professionals.

Although certain diseases, such as osteoporosis and diverticulosis, are very common in persons living in the western world, they are not universally present to the same degree and are now recognized as potentially preventable and clearly modifiable through diet modification. They are not to be considered normal or inevitable, but rather preventable. Hypertension, heart disease, and diabetes mellitus are just a few other examples of diseases that can be modified and even prevented. Unfortunately, most persons become concerned over problems only after they manifest later in life and perhaps even late in their course. Prevention is key and steps must be taken throughout life to maximize one's chances of staying healthy and functional. Simple changes in diet, lifestyle, and stress management can go a long way to improve our lifelong health and happiness.

There is often a fine line between things we do or fail to do that may accelerate the aging process and the development of disease. For example, smoking causes changes in lung function in a manner similar to the aging process; it can also lead to diseases such as emphysema, bronchitis, and even lung cancer. Exposure to excess UV light from the sun causes skin to prematurely wrinkle, but can also lead to skin cancers. Lack of calcium in the diet will result in our bones becoming less dense or demineralized. Over time, this will lead to the disease of osteoporosis and increase our risk of bone fractures, curvature of the spine, and immobility.

Medical science, however, still plays a key role in how successful we will age and in our ability to prevent as well as identify and treat illness early. Vaccinations now exist to prevent not only many of the childhood illnesses, but also that are capable of preventing influenza, tetanus, pneumococcal pneumonia, herpes zoster, and even cervical cancer.

The following is the Recommended Adult Immunization Schedule by Vaccine and Age Group. Please discuss this with your physician in order to keep up to date with latest recommendations. Vaccinations can prevent disease and they are not only for children!

Health screening can detect changes in blood sugar and blood pressure early so that treatment can be initiated prior to any end-organ damage. Certain cancers can be detected by simple screening tests and procedures including the PAP test, mammography, and colonoscopy. While in this case you are not preventing the disease, you are hopefully able to have treatment early and prevent the disease from progressing.

Attention to one's health is key if we are to live active and healthy lives and do whatever it takes to prevent disease from taking its toll on our lives. The

Vaccine	Age group		
	19–49	50–64	>65
Tetanus, diphtheria, pertussis(Td/Tdap)	Substitute 1-time dose of Tdap for Td booster; then boost with Td every 10 years		
Human papillomavirus (HPV)	3 doses for females through age 26 years; ideally given prior to starting sexual activity		
Influenza	1 dose annually		
Varicella[†]	2 doses		
Measles, mumps, rubella (MMR)	1 or 2 doses	1 dose	
Pneumococcal	1–2 doses[*,†]		1 dose
Hepatitis A[*,†]	2 doses		
Hepatitis B[*,†]	3 doses		
Meningococcal[*,†]	1 or more doses		
Zoster			1 dose

[*] Recommended if some other risk factor is present or in high risk group; discuss with your physician.
[†] Discuss with your physician.

importance of having a primary care physician who knows our health history, family dynamics, and insures proper health screening cannot be over emphasized. In this way, we also benefit from improved knowledge and available scientific data. For example, the U.S. Preventive Services Task Force (USPSTF) strongly recommends that physicians discuss the benefits and risks of using aspirin as a preventive medication for adults who are at increased risk for coronary heart disease. Men over the age of 40, postmenopausal women, and younger individuals with risk factors for coronary heart disease such as high blood pressure, diabetes, and/or smoking, are considered to be at increased risk and may wish to consider aspirin therapy. Insufficient sleep and excess stress are also known contributors to the development of disease and premature aging. Individuals with periodontal disease have also been shown to have an increased rate of heart disease, most likely because gum disease causes low-grade inflammation with systemic effects. Good dental hygiene with regular periodontal cleanings and treatment as necessary can help protect your heart as well as your teeth.

Proper diet, exercise and lifestyle modification can play a major role in helping to prevent many diseases from developing.

Examples of Age-Prevalent Illness

System	Disease
Central Nervous System	Dementia
	Depression
	Parkinsonism
	Stroke (CVA) or Transient Ischemic Attacks (TIA)
	Visual abnormalities (cataracts, macular degeneration, glaucoma)
	Hearing impairment
Cardiovascular System	Hypertension
	Ischemic heart disease
	Arrhythmia
	Congestive heart failure
	Peripheral vascular disease
	Varicose veins
	Aneurysms
	Aortic and Mitral Valve disease
Respiratory System	Chronic obstructive pulmonary disease
	Pneumonia
	Tuberculosis
	Bronchitis

Endocrine/Metabolic System	Diabetes Mellitus
	Hypothyroidism
	Electrolyte Abnormalities
	Gout
Gastrointestinal System	Hiatus hernia
	Dysphagia
	Constipation
	Fecal incontinence
	Diarrhea
	Malabsorption
	Ischemic colitis
	Irritable bowel syndrome
	Rectal prolapse
	Carcinoma of colon
Genitourinary System	Urinary tract infection
	Urinary incontinence
	Prostatic hypertrophy
	Renal insufficiency
	Prostate cancer
	Bladder cancer
	Impotence
Musculoskeletal System	Osteoporosis
	Osteoarthritis
	Paget's Disease
	Polymyalgia rheumatica
Hematological System	Anemia
	Multiple Myeloma
	Myelofibrosis
Autonomic Nervous System	Hypothermia
	Postural hypotension
Oral pharynx	Dental carries
	Periodontal diseases
	Dry mouth
Miscellaneous	Dehydration
	Foot problems
	Fractures
	Immobility
	Malnutrition
	Cancer
	Pressure Ulcers

4

Step 3: Recognize and Treat Problems Early

While we should all strive to do our very best to prevent the acceleration of our pre-determined "normal" aging process and to prevent the development of disease as best we can, for the foreseeable future, most of us still need to face the reality that some diseases may occur despite our best attempts to avoid them. Whether it is heart disease, cancer, high blood pressure, dementia, or some hormonal or neurological problem, diseases may present acutely or as subtle changes in the way we feel, think, or act. As we get older, many of the classic ways that diseases present earlier in life are no longer evident and in fact many diseases present in an atypical manner or with non-specific findings. These changes may result from normal aging phenomenon, such as the way our bodies can detect changes in the content of sugar or salt or adjust to changes in blood pressure. Chest pain may not be the first sign of a heart attack; shortness of breath is a more common presentation for many older persons. Pneumococcal pneumonia may not present in an older person with the usual fever, cough, and sputum production that is commonly seen in younger individuals; a urinary tract infection may first be heralded by a change in mental status, confusion, or even a fall with little or no symptoms related to the urinary tract.

Any change in one's usual state of health or feeling of well-being deserves to be evaluated and must not be underestimated or denied. While some of these may be a simple case of a 24-hour virus, a momentary feeling of despair, a response to a life event or even a change in the weather, these changes may also be the early stages of something more "serious". Failure to recognize that a problem may exist can delay beneficial treatment. Atypical and/or non-specific presentation of disease is clearly more common as one ages, but the principles are the same at any age. Putting off an evaluation or denying that a problem exists increases one's chances of having a more serious condition develop later on.

Studies have shown that certain groups of individuals are at higher risk of "under reporting" medical illness. These individuals include:

- "older" individuals who may not have the same warning signs they had in earlier life for similar problems. They may lack an awareness that they should seek assistance if they are not their in their "usual" state of health for whatever reason.
- persons who have difficulty with their mobility. This makes it harder for them to get to the physician and they may not want to be an inconvenience to family or friends and thus are not willing to ask for help.
- individuals who live alone and do not have the benefit of someone encouraging them to seek assistance.
- persons who have recently lost a loved one and who are at a higher risk of being depressed.
- individuals recently discharged from an acute-care hospital.

There are many reasons why one may "deny" that a problem exists or choose not to seek assistance. Perhaps there is some memory of a similar situation that affected a parent or grandparent or perhaps memory of a less than desirable outcome. It is important to be reminded that modern medicine has many treatments and options that were not even considered possible just a few years ago; the better we can keep informed of our options, the better we are in a position to choose wisely as to what is best for our specific needs and wishes.

It is so easy to put a problem "out of mind" if no one is there to urge us to seek help. It is frequently a family member, caregiver, or friend that has to urge one to seek assistance for a medical problem. It is easy to see how a person living alone is more likely to neglect something until much later in its course. The loss of a loved one is a difficult time for all and clearly increases one's risk of being depressed. Depressed individuals are more likely to neglect themselves in a similar way they might change their diet and activity. Despite the fact that one has just been in the hospital and received treatment, everyday individuals are re-admitted to the hospital with medication side-effects, infections that resulted from some contact or procedure performed during the hospital stay, or an inability to adhere to some regimen following the discharge.

Loved ones and friends would be wise to keep a look out for these "higher risk" individuals and offer support and encouragement as appropriate. The phrase "It takes a Village", popularized by Hilary Clinton, also applies in this case! The earlier we are able to recognize that a problem exists and initiate treatment, the less chance it has of becoming a life threatening problem or impact on one's future health and happiness.

Examples of Atypical and/or Non-Specific Presentations of Illness

Disease	Example
Pneumonia	Anorexia
	Confusion
	Normal pulse rate
	Normal body temperature
	Normal White Blood Cell Count
	Falls
Pulmonary Embolus	"Silent"
	Feelings of impending "doom"
Myocardial infarction	Shortness of breath
	Falls
	Weakness
	Absence of chest pain
	Anorexia
Acute Abdomen	Absence of any physical findings
	Weakness
	Confusion
Urinary tract infection	Confusion
	Falls
	No urinary tract symptoms
	Incontinence
	No rise in white blood cells
Parkinsonism	Falls
	Depression
	Slowness
Polymyalgia rheumatica	Aches/pains
	Lethargy
	Headache
	Weakness
Hyperthyroidism	Chest pain
	Palpitations
	Atrial fibrillation
	Shortness of breath
	Insomnia
	Weight loss
	Anorexia
	Absence of goiter

(*Continued*)

(*Continued*)

Disease	Example
Hypothyroidism	Depression
	Weakness
	Weight gain
	Confusion
	Anemia
	Vaginal bleeding
Depression	Dementia
	Slowing
	Weakness
	Constipation
	Weight loss
	Anorexia

There continues to be considerable debate and money spent on researching exactly how best to screen for various illnesses so that we can identify these as early in their course as possible. There are many organizations that have published guidelines to help physicians and individuals best determine what is cost-effective. The problem is not simple, however, as certain screening tests may have a "false positive" result, leading to additional testing and procedures that may in themselves result in problems. The U.S. Preventive Services Task Force (USPSTF) reports that the following screening tests are worth pursuing with benefits outweighing risks. You should discuss these with your physician if you have not already done so.

Men aged 35 and older and women aged 45 years and older should be screened for lipid disorders. Individuals who are at increased risk for coronary heart disease should be treated.

Men aged 20 to 35 years of age and women aged 20 to 45 years of age should be screened for lipid disorders if they have other risk factors for coronary heart disease.

While the USPSTF recommends against screening routinely for peripheral arterial disease, the Agency for Healthcare Research and Quality did suggest that physicians consider doing an ankle brachial index, a ratio of Doppler-recorded systolic blood pressures in the upper and lower extremities, as a simple and non-invasive method to assess and diagnosis peripheral arterial disease. An ankle-brachial index value of less than 0.90 is considered to be strongly associated with limitations in lower extremity function and physical activity and warrants further evaluation and possible treatment.

The USPSTF recommends one-time screening for abdominal aortic aneurysm by ultrasound testing in men aged 65 to 75 who have a history of having smoked anytime in their lives.

The USPSTF strongly recommends that all adults over the age of 18 have their blood pressure measured periodically and treated if elevated.

The USPSTF strongly recommends screening mammography, with or without clinical breast examination, every 1–2 years for women aged 40 and older. Follow-up testing and frequency should be individually determined based on findings.

The USPSTF strongly recommends regular screening for cervical cancer in women who have been sexually active and have a cervix. Many professional organizations recommend routine screening by age 18 or 21 for all women regardless of sexual history.

Women over the age of 65 who have had "adequate" recent screening and normal Pap test results may discontinue Pap testing. The American Cancer Society recommends stopping cervical cancer screening at age 70 for those who have had negative test results to date.

The USPSTF strongly recommends screening men and women 50 years of age and older for colorectal cancer. Potential screening options include home fecal occult blood testing, flexible sigmoidoscopy, combination of the two, colonoscopy, and double-contrast barium enema. The choice of specific screening should be based, they state, on patient preference, medical contraindications, patient's compliance, and available resources. Most physicians advocate for colonoscopy as the best test available at this time as it is thought to be the most sensitive and specific test for detecting cancer and large polyps. Tests should be repeated periodically with intervals based on the findings of the test. Talk to your physician about current recommendations as these will most likely change over time as newer tests become available.

Women aged 65 and older and women 60 years and older at increased risk for osteoporotic fractures should be screened for osteoporosis using a dual-photon densitometry measurement. Testing should be done for younger persons considered at greater risk of developing osteoporosis and thought to benefit from preventive treatment including persons on long-term steroid therapy and certain anti-convulsant medications.

While the USPSTF does not recommend for or against routine screening for prostate cancer using prostate specific antigen (PSA) or even the digital rectal examination, this remains a controversial area of research. The American College of Physicians suggests that patients and physicians individually discuss the pros and cons of testing, implications of a false positive test result, and that an approach be developed that is based on personal choice and understanding.

Other recommendations for screening include screening for alcohol misuse, asymptomatic bacteriuria in pregnant women, chlamydial infection in women, dental caries in pre-school children, depression in both men and women, diabetes mellitus in men and women, gonorrhea in women, hepatitis B virus infection in pregnant women, HIV in men and women, iron deficiency anemia in pregnant women, obesity, screening and counseling for tobacco use, and others.

Many professional organizations have their own list of recommendations and it is best to discuss these with your physician. For example, most physicians recommend a thorough eye examination every two years after age 50 with more frequent examinations if needed. In past years, an "annual history and physical examination" was part of routine medical care. Studies have not demonstrated that this is necessary for all persons without symptoms or already diagnosed disease and who are having the necessary preventive care and health screenings. After the age of 65, however, even if there are no apparent "problems" or health concerns, a comprehensive examination should, in my opinion, be performed every two years at a minimum and annually for those between 75 and 85 years of age. Individuals over the age of 85 should see their physician for a complete examination even if there is nothing obviously wrong or actively being treated every six months. With increasing age, there are just too many problems that may present "silently" or in a non-specific manner. The earlier we can recognize that something is not right, the better position we are in to treat them effectively. It is important that we all take responsibility for our own health and make sure that we are not only treating problems that we know of, but taking steps to recognize problems as early as possible through available screening tests and examinations.

5

Simple Steps You Can Take to Avoid Accelerating Your Aging Process

The Time to Start is NOW!

Avoid Environmental Hazards!

Environmental factors such as smog, excessive noise, sunlight, pollutants, and smoke are capable of accelerating our aging process and causing diseases that we otherwise would not likely get.

Smoking is a Health Hazard: It is Never Too Late to Stop!

Perhaps the best example of an environmental hazard that is under your control is cigarette smoking. Although our lungs normally undergo changes with age, these do not compromise our daily activities or health. Prolonged exposure to cigarette smoke, however, either actively or passively, can give a 50 year old person the lungs of an 80 year old. In addition, smoking increases one's chances of developing diseases such as emphysema, bronchitis, lung cancer and even stroke and heart disease.

"Smoking is the number one preventable cause of death among us today" we hear on the TV and radio. Yet, every day, countless numbers of our nation's youth start on this downward spiral to poor health and an accelerated aging process. While never starting to smoke is the best way to avoid problems, it is never too late to stop in order to see benefit. Research has clearly demonstrated that when a person stops smoking, the risk of heart disease and lung cancer drop dramatically over time. Non-smokers live on average at least four years longer than smokers, not to mention the improved quality of life that results from improved lung function and endurance and smoking related illness. Despite the wealth of anti-smoking literature, last year over 600 billion cigarettes were consumed. Lung cancer has overtaken breast cancer as the leading cause of cancer-related deaths among American women. Yes, as that popular cigarette company used to say in their ads: "You've come a long way baby!"

If every woman were to stop smoking today, within 18 to 24 months her lung function would return to normal, assuming no permanent damage had already occurred. Her risk of lung cancer, however, would not match that of her non-smoking counterpart for a full 15 years. We owe future generations the benefit of our knowledge regarding the evils of cigarette smoke, though for those who started smoking at an earlier time in life, all is not lost nor the situation helpless. Benefits have been demonstrated if one were to stop smoking at any age! Smoking cessation is within reach; however, it often takes more than just an "interest" in stopping. There are currently many medical treatment options available to assist someone to stop smoking. Nicotine is the culprit and until the body is able to overcome its addiction to this potent agent, a physical dependence will make stopping extremely difficult even for a person with great will power and motivation. Whether the nicotine replacement is by mouth or via a skin patch, it provides a systematic method of ridding nicotine dependence as it provides a scheduled dose reduction that weans one off the cigarettes. A centrally acting agent, buproprion, has been demonstrated to help reduce the urge to smoke with several studies demonstrating an even higher success rate than nicotine replacement gum or patches. This also has the added advantage that if someone were to lapse and take a cigarette while they were trying to stop smoking all together, they would not suffer the potential side-effects from excess nicotine that would occur if one were using a nicotine substitute. What works for one person may not be as useful for another — individual problems require individual solutions. Some individuals are able to stop smoking "cold turkey" with nothing more than strong will and good intentions. Being a "smoker", however, is a lifetime label, much like other addictions. The urge to smoke commonly arises when someone is surrounded by others who smoke. As with most addictions, prevention may require an adjustment to lifestyle and habits and avoiding those things that serve as triggers. A diary may be necessary to help link situations that led to a relapse with precipitating situations and/or events.

Unfortunately, many persons who smoke do so for reasons other than physical dependency. Some individuals have what is commonly referred to as an oral fixation, using the presence of something in the mouth as a way to provide a calming effect. Perhaps this relates to some childhood technique our parents taught us or a self-learned behavior or habit; subconscious coping mechanisms are not uncommon and must be dealt with head on! Chewing gum is one way people can often cope with this need rather than reach for a cigarette; caution is advised, however, not to substitute food or snacks as another way of appeasing an oral fixation. Weight gain is often reported in those who stop smoking. While many argue it is the substitution of one addiction, food, for another, cigarettes, and in certain circumstances it is, the situation is not so simple. Studies have demonstrated a transient decline in metabolic activity upon smoking cessation. This reduction in metabolism will reduce one's caloric expenditure and can result in weight gain even if one were to maintain exactly the same number of calories one consumed prior to stopping smoking. Fortunately, this change in metabolism appears to be transient. The difference, however, is that now you will have a new lease on life and additional quality years to look forward to. Increasing exercise upon smoking cessation is one way to counteract the tendency to gain wait. Support groups also have proven beneficial and should be used if one finds stopping "too difficult" or the urge to start smoking again too strong. Unfortunately, much like the alcoholic, one is always a smoker even when one is no longer smoking. I have heard of people "smoking in their dreams" many years after stopping the actual act of smoking. Once again, the best way to stop is to never start — a good lesson to teach our children and future generations.

Smoking has been demonstrated to not only have undesirable consequences on the person who smokes, but also to anyone exposed to the cigarette smoke. This has been referred to as passive smoking. Children whose parents smoke have more respiratory infections and asthma. Years of "secondary" exposure to smoke has also been implicated in a higher rate of developing lung cancer even in those individuals who have never smoked themselves.

The choice is yours to make. The benefits are scientifically proven and without a doubt will benefit not only you but also those around you.

Dangers of Ultra-Violet Rays/Sun Exposure

Ultra-violet rays from the sun or from artificial sources may give you that healthy-looking tan which may be attractive in the short term, but beware! These rays are also capable of accelerating the aging of your skin and will increase skin wrinkling and dryness. In addition, those who worship the sun in pursuit of that bronzed outdoor look risk developing skin cancer later in life. Skin cancer is the fastest growing cancer today. Not only does this likely result from changes in lifestyle and an increased amount of leisure time spent in the sun, but also may result as our natural protection from harmful UV rays, the ozone layer, dissipates, leading to increasing amounts of these harmful rays reaching the earth and our skin. Furthermore, lifetime exposure to excessive sunlight may damage our vision. Ultraviolet rays can damage the cornea, the lens, and even the retina. Cataracts, or clouding of the lens of the eye and macular degeneration, destruction of cells in that part of the eye responsible for our best vision, are increasingly common and major threats as we age.

Sunburn, an inflammation caused by the ultraviolet rays of the sun, results in damage to the cells in the outer layer of the skin and toughens it. Even worse, studies have demonstrated that even one case of severe sunburn early in life increases one's risk of developing melanoma, the most serious and often deadly form of skin cancer many years later.

Prevention of these problems can be as simple as wearing a hat to block the harmful rays from reaching the skin and sunglasses capable of screening out harmful ultra-violet rays. While a baseball cap provides a brim that protects the face, it does little to shield the back of the neck and ears, common sites for the development of skin cancers. Choosing a proper protective hat is essential to good health.

Sunglasses that provide dark lenses are not all created equal with some actually being worse than wearing no sunglasses at all despite a feeling of comfort. Under dark conditions, the pupil, or the opening into the eye, dilates to allow more light to penetrate into the nerve layer or retina that lines the back of the eye and allows sight to occur.

Unless the lens of the sunglasses filters out harmful UV light, you can see how simply wearing a dark lens can be harmful despite a feeling that one is protected. UV rays enter the eye without any apparent notice, much like the observer of a total eclipse of the sun risks going blind as the UV rays will continue to enter the eye and damage the retina despite one's ability to look directly at the sun in these rare circumstances.

Protection against wrinkles and skin cancer is easily within reach by using sunscreen and common sense. Not all sun screening lotions or creams are equal and one should make sure that both UV A and B are blocked. While there are individual SPF numbers assigned to all sun screening lotions, this only provides a guide as to how often the lotion must be re-applied in order to work and not how effective they are in blocking the UV rays. They also will differ in terms of their effects on the skin with some blocking pores more than others and causing acne; some have "soothing" additives such as aloe vera and may be better for individuals with dry skin. We have indeed come a long way from the time when "sun lotions" were to help one maximize the effects of the sun to our current thinking that exposure to UV light should be limited and UV light blocking lotions used whenever sun exposure is likely to occur.

Some individuals obtain their "tanned" look by going to a tanning salon and being exposed to what some claim is a safer, more limited, spectrum of UV light. Even though the time of exposure is usually quite limited and the rays chosen are perhaps less damaging than the full spectrum of UV light that comes directly from the sun, these treatments may also lead to premature wrinkling and even skin cancer and in my opinion are best avoided. Once again, the choice is yours to make!

Avoid Noise Pollution

Minor hearing loss, particularly for high frequency sounds, is a normal condition of aging. Men appear to be affected more than women but in itself, these normal changes rarely cause interference with one's daily routine such as listening to the radio, TV, or hearing conversations in a crowed room. Exposure to "loud" noises earlier in life, however, can accelerate the loss of hearing to the point that certain sounds may compete with voices as annoying background "noise", creating difficulty in interpreting what is being said or result in speech that sounds "mumbled". Loud "rock" music, subway and aircraft noise, and gunshot sounds are just a few sounds that are capable of damaging our hearing, especially if the exposure is prolonged or of extreme nature. We have a society of young individuals who flourish listening to MP3 players. Parents should educate their children about the potential harms of excessive noise and do whatever possible to limit the loudness of the music being played for hours on end.

An estimated 20 million Americans have hearing problems. The Federal Occupational Safety and Health Administration (OSHA) has set 85 decibels as the level above which the potential exists for hearing damage. This represents the approximate loudness of conversation on a noisy bus. Not only is loudness a factor, but also the duration of exposure. It has been said that as few as two hours of exposure to 100 decibels results in some degree of permanent hearing loss. Headphones on a radio can often exceed this limit and thus concern for those who utilize earphones to any significant degree. One hundred and twenty decibels, such as the sound emanating directly from the front of speakers at a rock concert may result in immediate damage to our functional hearing.

Prevention is the best cure! Keep sounds to a minimum and use earplugs or protective headgear when excessive exposure is impossible to avoid. These preventive measures can help preserve our hearing as we age.

Hearing loss occurs in two forms. The first is referred to as a conduction defect and can occur for a number of reasons including damage to the auditory or 8th cranial nerve, or the delicate bones within the middle part of the ear, the hammer, anvil, and stirrup. Damage may occur if these bones become calcified or develop cholesterol deposits that interfere with their functioning. Sounds appear along the entire hearing spectrum to be diminished and the individual will not be able to hear sounds below a critical threshold of decibels, a measure of loudness. Normal conversation occurs at approximately 50 decibels and whispers between 20 and 30. This is the easiest type of hearing deficit to correct as anything that will magnify sounds will improve one's ability to hear and function. Infrared devices are sold with headphones that make sounds louder to the wearer while filtering out competing outside sounds. Whether used for watching television, listening to a speaker in a crowded auditorium, or going to the movies or a play, this technology has become much more widely available and the cost less prohibitive. Hearing aids may also be used to augment sounds for a person in need at all times.

The more common problem causing hearing difficulties results from a change in one's ability to hear certain frequencies of sound, whether they be high, medium, or low. Presbyaccusis, a form of neurosensory hearing loss, is a term that refers to the high frequency hearing deficit that accompanies the normal aging process. If accelerated, one has difficulty hearing when there is more than one source of sound or speech occurring in a crowded, noisy room. High frequency hearing is necessary to hear consonants; these letters have been shown to be essential to understanding someone talking clearly; speech may sound "mumbled" to a person with high frequency hearing loss. Another problem results because many background sounds are in the high frequency range, such as fluorescent lights, air-conditioners, motors, among many other everyday occurrences. These sounds may now sound more like a "roar" or a "buzz" to the person with a high frequency hearing loss than the actual sound one was previously familiar with. This may interfere with hearing what is being said; merely making sounds louder will not solve the problem as the abnormal sounds will now also be louder and much more problematic. This problem is usually remedied by the use of a specially designed hearing aid following an assessment and analysis of the hearing problem. An audiogram, or mapping of sounds of various levels of loudness (decibels) and frequencies, is done by an audiologist, a specialist in hearing problems. Based on these findings, a hearing aid can be created to make certain sounds along the spectrum louder or lower and thus improve one's ability to hear the spoken word. Noises are reduced and speech is clearer even in areas with competing sounds.

It is amazing to see how many people have re-directed their interests based on a hearing loss without even being aware that they have done so. Not only may individuals choose to no longer go to a movie or play, but studies have reported reduced participation in group activities; depression is also a major coincident problem.

Unfortunately, many older persons who tried a hearing aid years ago claim that it did not help them to hear better and are reluctant to try again. Older hearing aids not only were larger, but they were less able to adjust frequencies and often background sounds became even more problematic. We are fortunate to live in a time of rapid technological advancement. Modern hearing aids are now so small that they can fit within the opening of the ear itself and can be individually crafted to selectively increase or decrease specific frequencies to correct for individual problems and return the specific frequency hearing that was lost.

Sometimes, the ear plays tricks on us and we develop a condition known as tinnitus, a problem more common with hearing loss. This occurs more commonly in persons who have already lost high frequency hearing and a buzz, hiss, or whooshing sound is present even in complete silence. At times this noise can be maddening and result in depression and even thoughts of suicide. Medical help is available and new technology is promising though the best way to avoid this problem is to practice prevention and do whatever necessary to preserve hearing throughout life.

Most importantly, while prevention is key to preserving one's hearing, even those with functional hearing loss can receive help and should be encouraged to seek an assessment by a qualified audiologist. Neurosensory hearing loss due to the loss of critical nerve cells in the inner ear that send the message to the brain by way of the 8th cranial nerve may not be reversible if the damage to the "hair cells" has already occurred; its further decline, however, can often be prevented and usually functional hearing can be restored with the use of hearing aids and assistive devices. Sometimes, the solution is simple, e.g. wax that has impacted the ear canal and is preventing the ear drum from detecting sound waves. In other cases, fluid has accumulated in the middle ear and this too can affect the way our ears conduct sounds to the brain. In any case, functional hearing loss should not be considered a "normal consequence" of growing old!

6

Eat a Healthy Diet to Promote Wellness and Prevent Disease

Although eating is an activity everyone should know a great deal about, many persons fail to eat a nutritionally balanced diet. In fact, many individuals do not even know if what they are eating is healthy or what they might eat to maximize their aging process and health. Many people eat to excess or fail to eat basic requirements necessary for health. Malnutrition is not something observed only in third world countries. It can result whenever there is a deficiency or excess of a specific required nutrient or calories. Our daily intake of nutrients should provide the body with the basic materials it needs to stay healthy and function normally. Besides an essential amount of proteins, carbohydrates, and fats, we must ensure an adequate intake of vitamins, minerals and trace elements.

What is most worrisome is the growing number of individuals who are obese. Over 30% of the US population is currently considered to be significantly over-weight and at increased risk of developing obesity associated problems such as heart disease, diabetes, arthritis, sleep-apnea, strokes and hypertension, among others. This is also a growing problem in other parts of the world that appears to correlate with the rise in fast-food establishments, busy work schedules, and increased portion size.

There are numerous reasons that have been suggested to help explain this apparent epidemic that is also increasingly affecting our children. These include portion size increasing in recent decades; fast-food becoming more of a staple in the American diet with many more families having two income earners, each with less time to devote to household chores and meal preparation; the proliferation of snack foods with high concentrations of "refined" sugars; the greater focus on mass transit and automobile travel; the reduction in daily physical activity, and others.

Certain foods may have protective effects against heart disease and cancer while others may actually promote illness. The trick is finding the "right food" that is nutritionally sound and that you like. In general, red meat and food with high fat content are most worrisome. Research has shown that animal fat and animal protein may pre-dispose one to the development of certain cancers including rectal and colon, breast, and prostate. The prostate cancer death rate, for example, is five times higher in the United States and in northern Europe than it is in Hong Kong, Iran, Turkey and Japan where diets emphasize more vegetables, grains, beans, cereals, and fruits. Fat in the diet also pre-disposes one to heart disease. We are learning more each day but there is already a wealth of data available to help us make wiser choices when planning our diets. Omega-3 fatty acids, cholesterol, anti-oxidants, trans-fats are just a few of the terms we need to master and understand before we can choose a healthy diet plan that will "work" and promote a more successful aging process and a lifetime of wellbeing.

The Role of Antioxidants in Promoting a More Successful Aging Process

Antioxidants have received a great deal of attention in recent years. Hundreds of studies in animals, cells, and humans have demonstrated a beneficial effect of antioxidants in protecting against the harmful "oxidation" process that potentially can harm every cell, organ, and tissue in the body. Oxygen is ubiquitous and is essential to life. However, if the oxygen molecule looses one of its two electrons, it is transformed into a "singlet oxygen" and circulates in the body trying to either donate or steal an electron. In doing this, it sets up a series of reactions in the body that if left unchecked produce the hydroxyl radical, a potent oxidant and cause of illness and cellular destruction. While our body has certain enzymes that help eliminate these dangerous substances, it is possible that we may have just too many to handle and without the additional help of antioxidants, harm is inevitable. In fact, this is one theory as to why we "age" and develop so many degenerative diseases later in life. This process has been referred to as the "Free Radical Theory on Aging" as these superoxide substances are also referred to as "free radicals". This theory as to aging was first proposed in 1956 by Dr. Denham Harman who went on to found the American Aging Association. I was fortunate to be involved in this organization, eventually being elected its President.

Antioxidants can be derived from certain foods in the diet or obtained from supplemental vitamins and minerals such as Vitamin E, Vitamin A, selenium and Vitamin C. In general, foods that are deep purple, red, green or orange have the greatest amount of antioxidants. The carotenoids and anthocyanins provide color to foods that contain significant amounts of antioxidants. Foods rich in antioxidants include almonds, berries, citrus fruits, carrots, spinach, tomatoes, and bell peppers, among others. Green tea and dark chocolate have also been suggested as having beneficial effects due to their relatively high antioxidant properties from flavonoids. Green tea comes in many varieties but if used appropriately and brewed fresh, it can provide a safe and satisfying way to augment the intake of antioxidants. Dark chocolate, while also rich in flavonoids, has the added problem of being relatively high in calories.

New investigations have demonstrated that low serum/plasma levels of carotenoids are independently associated with poor skeletal muscle strength and impaired physical performance in older individuals. Low levels of serum/plasma carotenoids have also been associated with the development of insulin resistance and diabetes, both age-prevalent disorders with potentially serious health consequences. Epidemiological data from populations that adhere to the Mediterranean diet, characterized by a high intake of fruits, vegetables and whole grains and a relatively low intake of red meat and saturated fats, have demonstrated not only lower circulating levels of the inflammatory marker, IL-6, but also reduced rates of cardiovascular disease and certain cancers as compared to individuals on other forms of diet.

The following is a partial listing of some of the health benefits claimed from foods that are rich in both color and antioxidants in addition to the benefits listed above. Unfortunately, most of these claims come from uncontrolled studies or are based on data from populations eating large quantities of these foods as compared to those who do not. While additional studies are clearly needed, most of the following foods are worth considering as part of one's daily intake of fruits and vegetables.

Deep green-cruciferous vegetables such as broccoli have been reported to help prevent colon cancer. Spinach and kale are not only rich in antioxidants, but are also good sources of calcium and help promote bone health. Kale has been reported to help protect against macular degeneration, the leading cause of blindness in older individuals.

Red-Tomatoes are rich in lycopene and are thought to help protect against prostate and cervical cancers. They also are rich in Vitamin C, an antioxidant necessary to maintain healthy skin and connective tissue.

Orange/yellow-squash, carrots, sweet potatoes, and yams are thought to promote healthy lungs and help protect against skin cancers.

Deep blue/purple-eggplant, plums, blueberries, blackberries (including strawberries, raspberries, and cherries) reportedly lower the risk of heart disease and have been even suggested as a way to help improve memory. Red grapes have been associated with lower rates of heart disease and even lung cancer.

Interestingly, recently published well controlled studies that have evaluated the effects of taking supplemental doses of vitamins with potent anti-oxidant properties in dosages greater than that considered to be the daily requirement and through non-dietary sources, have failed to demonstrate benefits in reducing heart disease and cancer. Whether dietary sources act in a different way or the higher amounts obtained through supplements exceed that required for benefit are not currently known. A study conducted in 2004 in Denmark on persons who already had been diagnosed with esophageal, gastric, colorectal, pancreatic or liver cancer failed to demonstrate any benefit from the use of any combination of beta carotene, selenium, Vitamins A, C, and E. In fact, there was a 6% higher death rate noted for those who took the antioxidant containing vitamins. It is possible that individuals taking these agents may not have adhered to more conventional treatments and thus the higher death rate. This was also a study conducted on individuals who already had serious and life-threatening cancer. One must be cautious when trying to interpret the literature. Additional research is clearly needed as the available data from both human and animal studies remain conflicted.

7

The Role of Vitamins in Promoting Successful Aging

A simple multivitamin cannot replace eating well; however, it may be necessary to supplement diets that fail to provide sufficient food choices or are limited in one specific food group. In general, individuals eating less than 1,500 calories a day benefit from taking a daily vitamin and mineral supplement as their choice of foods is simply too limited to insure adequate amounts of all required nutrients. Many persons who consume higher amounts of calories, however, may still fall short in certain required areas. This is particularly a problem for individuals who prefer to exclude entire classes of food, such as vegans or those on "fad" diets. While a simple daily vitamin formulated to provide 100% of the daily requirements rarely causes harm, mega vitamins are not to be taken without considerable thought as vitamin toxicities can be life threatening and data suggest that at least some of them may have adverse effects.

Vitamins are in one of two forms, either water or fat soluble. Most water soluble vitamins taken to excess are excreted in the urine; while side-effects are rare, they may still produce significant illness. Vitamin C, for example, competes in the kidney with oxalate. If you happen to have an excessive amount of oxalate in the urine either due to a genetic predisposition or excessive intake from food, such as eating large quantities of rhubarb, taking as little as 250 mg of Vitamin C may lead to the formation of calcium oxalate kidney stones. Those considering taking doses of water soluble vitamins in excess of the established RDA should seek guidance from a knowledgeable physician or registered dietitian.

Fat soluble Vitamins A, D, E and K, are stored in the body's fat and accumulate at higher concentrations as we age due to a change in body composition and increased size of the fat deposits. The amount of fat soluble vitamins contained in the usual daily vitamin is low enough to cause no harm in the majority of persons taking them. If taken to excess, however, Vitamin A can cause a disease referred to as pseudo-tumor cerebrae, a disorder that mimics symptoms of a brain tumor. Many a polar explorer fell prey to this illness due to toxic levels of Vitamin A found in polar bear livers, a source of food in a time of starvation. Fortunately, carotene, a precursor of Vitamin A and a common source of this important vitamin does not have the same toxicity; excessive intake, however, may lead to a harmless yellowish hue to the skin and depending on whether you believe the data, may increase one's risk of developing illness. Excess Vitamin D can lead to a higher than normal level of calcium that at times can be life threatening.

Clearly a balance is necessary as each is essential to good health and proper functioning, yet if taken to excess, can result in illness and even death. A recent randomized, double-blind, placebo-controlled study concluded that individuals who took a multivitamin had a lower level of C-reactive protein. This has significance since elevated C-reactive protein levels appear to serve as a marker of systemic inflammation and is considered to be a risk factor for the development of cardiovascular disease and diabetes. Individual studies have linked lower C-reactive protein levels with higher concentrations of pyridoxal 5'-phosphate, a circulating form of Vitamin B6, in the plasma. Ascorbic acid (Vitamin C) and alpha-tocopherol (Vitamin E) have also been favorably linked to lower levels of C-reactive protein as has the intake of foods rich in omega-3 fatty acids.

The following is a more detailed discussion of the major water soluble and fat soluble vitamins and their major characteristics, benefits and risks.

Fat Soluble Vitamins

Vitamin A

Vitamin A consists of a group of compounds essential for proper vision, growth, cellular development, reproduction, and proper functioning of the immune system. Retinol, retinaldehyde, and retinoic acid are naturally occurring compounds that contain some degree of Vitamin A activity. A large number of synthetic compounds also have Vitamin A activity and are collectively referred to as retinoids. While some of these compounds may provide protection from deficiency states that may result from an inadequate intake of Vitamin A in the diet, they may not provide complete protection. For example, retinoic acid taken in the diet does not protect against night blindness or reproductive dysfunction.

Vitamin A is obtained through the diet by consuming pre-formed retinoids that have Vitamin A activity. These are usually found in animal products and foods rich in carotenoid precursors of Vitamin A such as beta-carotene, alpha-carotene, and cryptoxanthin. These latter products are found in plants as well as in some animal fats. There are over 500 carotenoids found naturally of which only 50 or so are precursors of retinol and thus considered to have pro-Vitamin A activity. All-trans Beta-carotene is the most active Vitamin A product on a weight basis.

Pre-formed Vitamin A is present in foods of animal origin in the form of retinyl ester. This is hydrolyzed in the small intestine to form retinol and carotenoids. Most absorbed Beta-carotene is converted to retinol and then to retinyl esters in the mucosal cells of the intestine. These retinyl esters and carotenoids are taken up from the blood as it passes through the liver and stored in the form of retinyl esters. The storage efficiency of ingested Vitamin A in the liver is more than 50% with the liver containing approximately 90% of the body's stores of the vitamin.

Vitamin A Deficiency

Vitamin A deficiency is found most commonly in children under the age of 5 and is usually due to an insufficient dietary intake. Deficiency may also result from insufficient absorption of fats by the intestine. This is usually accompanied by intestinal problems such as diarrhea. Clinical features of a deficiency of Vitamin A commonly include night blindness and conjunctival and/or corneal xerosis, ulceration, and sometimes liquefaction. These ocular manifestations are referred to collectively as xerophthalmia. Keratomalacia is the term for irreversible corneal lesions associated with partial or total blindness and may also result from a Vitamin A deficiency.

Other findings may also include a loss of appetite, hyperkeratosis, increased susceptibility to infections, and changes in the cell structure of peripheral cells of the respiratory tract and other organs.

Vitamin A Excess

Excessive intake of Vitamin A, either acutely or chronically may result in numerous toxic effects including headache, vomiting, diplopia or double-vision, alopecia or areas of baldness, dryness of the mucous membranes, bone abnormalities and liver damage. There is also a potential for spontaneous abortions and birth defects including malformations of the skull, face, heart, and central nervous system observed in fetuses of women ingesting even "therapeutic doses" of 13-cis retinoic acid during the first trimester of pregnancy (0.5 to 1.5 mg/kg). Large daily doses of retinyl esters or retinol, greater than 6,000 RE or 20,000 IU, may cause similar abnormalities.

Carotenoids, even when ingested in very large doses for weeks to years have until recently been considered non-toxic. This is due to their significantly lower efficiency of absorption at high doses and limited conversion to Vitamin A in the intestine, liver, and other organs. Carotenoids, however, when taken in large doses for weeks are absorbed in sufficient amounts to color the fat tissue including the subcutaneous fat. This will turn the skin, especially the palms of the hands and soles of the feet, to a yellowish hue. This coloration will gradually disappear when the high intake is discontinued.

It is important to note, however, that Vitamin A supplementation in the form of beta-carotene may have undesirable effects. This method of providing Vitamin A was studied in the Carotene and Retinol Efficacy Trial to assess the effect these forms of Vitamin A had on a variety of end points, including cancer risk. While certain benefits were described, the use of mega-supplements of beta-carotene, but not retinol, were associated with an increased risk of dying from lung cancer. A 1994 study conducted in Finland with smokers taking 20 mg a day of beta-carotene demonstrated an 18% higher incidence of lung cancer as compared to those who did not take this. In 1996, a study examined the effects of taking beta carotene and Vitamin A in a population who were smokers and individuals exposed to asbestos, two major causes of lung cancer. These individuals had a 28% greater risk of developing lung cancer and a 26% higher risk of dying from heart disease as compared to those not taking the supplements. In 2002, a study involving more than 72,000 nurses revealed that individuals who consumed the highest amount of Vitamin A through diet, multivitamins, and supplements, in doses above that which is recommended, had a 48% greater risk of suffering a hip fracture as compared to the nurses taking lower amounts. The Institute of Medicine does not recommend beta-carotene supplements for the general population beyond what one can obtain through a well-balanced diet or simple multi-vitamin.

Dietary Sources of Vitamin A

The richest sources of preformed retinol are liver and fish liver oils. Significant quantities can also be found in whole and fortified milk and in eggs. Data from the second (1976–1980) National Health and Nutrition Examination Survey (NHANES11) indicated that the major contributors of Vitamin A or pro-Vitamin A in the American diet came from liver, carrots, eggs, vegetable-based soups, and whole milk products. Fortified foods also contribute to dietary intake of Vitamin A with approximately 1/3 of the US population currently reported to take supplements of Vitamin A in one form or another. Less than one-third of total Vitamin A activity in the diet is derived from carotenoids.

Recommended Daily Allowance

The current RDA for Vitamin A is 1,000 micrograms (3,000 IU) for men and 800 micrograms (2,330 IU) for women. The amount of Beta-carotene necessary to meet the Vitamin A requirement of adult men is approximately twice that of retinol. The Institute of Medicine does not recommend carotene supplements for the general population or Vitamin A intake beyond the amount suggested above.

Vitamin D

Vitamin D is also referred to as calciferol and is essential for the proper formation of the bony skeleton and for proper balance of the key minerals, calcium and phosphorous. Exposure of the skin to ultraviolet light is necessary in order to form Vitamin D3, otherwise known as cholecalciferol, from its precursor, 7-dehydrocholesterol. D2, or ergocalciferol is another form of Vitamin D and is the product of the ultraviolet light-induced conversion of ergosterol in plants. Once formed, D3 circulates throughout the body. When D3 passes through the liver it becomes 1.5 times more potent when a hydroxyl (OH) group is added to form 25-hydroxy D3. This compound continues to circulate through the body and is once again fortified as it passes through the kidney and another change occurs as a second hydroxyl group is added, this time to the 1 position of D3 to form 1,25 dihydroxy Vitamin D3. This final compound is now 5 times more potent than the original vitamin that began in the skin.

Vitamin D status is usually assessed by measuring levels of 25-hydroxy Vitamin D3 and 1,25 dihydroxy Vitamin D3. The average value of 25 hydroxy Vitamin D3 ranges from approximately 25 to 30 ng/ml with the current recommended level being at least 30 ng/ml; the concentration of 1,25 di-hydroxy Vitamin D3 under normal circumstances is between 15–45 pg/ml in healthy adults. There appears to be little seasonal variation in the concentration of 1,25 di-hydroxy Vitamin D3, though levels of 25-OH Vitamin D3 may rise during summer months in relation to sun exposure.

One international unit (IU) of Vitamin D3 is defined as the activity of 0.025 micrograms of cholecalciferol in bioassays that use rats and chicks. This results in cholecalciferol having a biological activity of 40 IU/microgram. As stated above, the activity of 25-hydroxy Vitamin D3 and 1,25 di-hydroxy Vitamin D3 is 1.5 and 5 times, respectively greater than that of Vitamin D3.

Vitamin D is added to many dairy products at a concentration of 10 micrograms of cholecalciferol (400 IU) per quart. Human milk contains between 0.63 and 1.25 micrograms of cholecalciferol per liter. Eggs and butter also contain some Vitamin D.

Individuals regularly exposed to sunlight and without specific problems that may interfere with normal Vitamin D metabolism are not considered to have a dietary requirement for Vitamin D. Since so many individuals do not achieve a normal balance, however, the RDA for adults has been placed at 5 micrograms (200 IU) per day. In aged individuals and those with osteoporosis, the recommended daily allowance has been suggested between 400–800 IU with some individuals requiring even greater amounts to achieve the desired blood level of 25-OH Vitamin D3 of between 30–45 pg/ml.

Vitamin D deficiency is characterized by inadequate mineralization of the skeleton. In children, this results in the disease known as rickets and causes skeletal deformities such as a "bowing" of the knees and "knobs" over the ribs. In adults this problem is referred to as osteomalacia and may be confused with another major problem affecting the skeleton, e.g. osteoporosis as both may be associated with a higher risk of skeletal fractures. Osteomalacia is commonly associated with micro-fractures and skeletal pain as the disease progresses. Weakness and falls have also been associated with Vitamin D deficiency states as well as depression. In a study conducted as part of the Longitudinal Aging Study in Amsterdam, Netherlands, 1,282 subjects aged 65–95 were studied; 26 were found to have a major depressive disorder and 169, minor depression. Levels of 25 (OH) Vitamin D were significantly lower in those with depression as compared to those without and were consistent even when possible variables were taken into account such as history of smoking, co-existing illness, and body mass index. There was also a correlation made between depression and levels of parathyroid hormone (PTH) with highest levels found in those with the most significant depression. It is well known that there is an inverse relationship between Vitamin D levels and levels of PTH. Hypocalcemia and hypophosphetemia may also be noted in persons with Vitamin D deficient states. Recent studies have also linked low levels of Vitamin D with an increased risk of falling.

Vitamin D deficiency may not only result from diets that contain inadequate quantities of Vitamin D. Malabsorption of fats may lead to Vitamin D deficiency as Vitamin D is a fat-soluble vitamin. Changes in Vitamin D metabolism may result from the use of medications such as Phenobarbital and Dilantin.

Under general conditions, Vitamin D can be produced in adequate amounts if the skin is exposed to a sufficient amount of sunlight or artificial ultraviolet radiation. Of course, the amount of Vitamin D synthesized through this mechanism will depend on the amount of the skin exposed, time of exposure, as well as the season of the year and the wavelength of the ultraviolet light on the skin. We have become increasingly aware of the dangers of excessive exposure to sunlight and there has been greater avoidance of sun exposure, use of "protective" clothing, and sunscreens. These will limit the ability of the body to produce sufficient quantities of Vitamin D. Furthermore, skin from elderly individuals is less able to synthesize Vitamin D3 due to age related changes. For these reasons, many individuals fail to maintain an adequate amount of Vitamin D in the circulation. Of course, individuals who are dark skinned require a longer exposure to ultraviolet light to achieve the same effect; individuals with kidney and/or liver disease will be additionally effected and less able to metabolize Vitamin D3 into its more potent forms.

Vitamin D is potentially toxic, especially in young children. Excessive intake of Vitamin D may result in hypercalcemia and hypercalciuria, an excessive amount of calcium being excreted into the urine. These findings can lead to the deposition of calcium in soft tissues and irreversible renal and even cardiovascular damage. While no specific amount of Vitamin D can be set as the minimum for toxicity, many persons run the risk of becoming toxic if they exceed an intake of 45 micrograms (1,800 IU) of cholecalciferol per day for a prolonged period of time.

Vitamin E

Vitamin E is considered essential for normal reproductive and neuro-muscular health. First discovered in 1922, Vitamin E has received much recent attention as a potent anti-oxidant. Deficiency rarely occurs, though such states have been described in premature infants and those with fat malabsorption. Of note, malabsorption must persist for 5–10 years before a deficiency state results.

Two Vitamin E compounds are found naturally in plants. Tocopherol, characterized by a ring system and a long, saturated side chain, can be found in four sub-types. The tocotrienols have an unsaturated side chain. The most active form of Vitamin E is alpha-tocopherol, the most widely distributed form in nature.

The activity of 1 mg of the acetate form of alpha-tocopherol has been defined as equivalent to 1 IU of Vitamin E. Although too complicated to discuss in detail, naturally occurring Vitamin E is referred to as alpha-tocopherol and is also designated as RRR-alpha-tocopherol. Synthetic compounds of Vitamin E are designated all-rac-alpha tocopherol and have approximately 74% of the activity of the naturally occurring compound. Since there are also three other naturally occurring types of tocopherol, these must also be considered in one's total intake with an appropriate adjustment in activity; beta-tocopherol, for example is half as potent and gamma-tocopherol only one-tenth as potent as alpha-tocopherol.

As stated above, tocopherols serve as chemical antioxidants and prevent oxidative damage that result from free radicals. Due to the fact that Vitamin E is ubiquitously present in cell membranes and is associated with polyunsaturated fatty acids that are present in phospholipids found in the body, a deficiency state may lead to cell damage and eventually neurological symptoms. Other anti-oxidants that exist in the body include selenium, a component of the enzyme glutathione peroxidase, and Vitamin C, or ascorbic acid.

Only 20–80% of alpha-tocopherol is absorbed from the intestine and normal biliary and pancreatic function are essential. As the dose of Vitamin E increases, the body is less able to absorb it. Vitamin E is secreted into the lymph system in chylomicrons. These are taken up into the liver, and are subsequently secreted into the blood along with very low density lipoproteins (VLDL's). As these VLDL's are metabolized, tocopherol is transferred to low density lipoproteins (LDL's) and high density lipoproteins (HDL's). Binding of alpha-tocopherol has been found in the liver and red blood cells. Tissues with high lipid concentrations have the highest concentration of tocopherol, such as the liver and adrenal glands. When expressed on the basis of lipid content, however, most tissues have been found to have similar levels.

Normal blood concentrations of total tocopherols in adult men and women range from 0.6 to 1.2 mg/dl. Because alpha-tocopherol is carried by lipoproteins, the plasma lipid content can influence its concentration.

Compared to other fat soluble vitamins, Vitamin E is relatively non-toxic when consumed orally in recommended doses. Oral doses between 100 and 400 mg/day are well tolerated and considered safe; some argue that doses as high as 800 mg/day are also acceptable and without risk. As stated previously, deficiency states, while rare have been associated with neurological findings and when plasma Vitamin E is considerably below normal, red blood cells may become susceptible to excessive hemolysis or breakage due to changes in the red blood cell's structural membrane.

The tocopherol content of foods varies greatly depending on its processing, method of storage, and the method of food preparation. The richest sources of tocopherol in the US diet are the common vegetable oils, including soybean, corn, cottonseed, and safflower oil and products that are made from them such as margarine and shortening. The exact ratio of the various forms of tocopherol will vary between foods. Wheat germ is particularly high in Vitamin E as are nuts and green leafy vegetables.

The average intake of Vitamin E and alpha-tocopherol among men and women aged 19–50 years is 9.8 mg and 7.1 mg, respectively. As one increases the intake of polyunsaturated fatty acids (PUFA) in the diet, however, there is a need for higher amounts of Vitamin E. For this reason, requirements vary greatly and are thought to vary between 5 and 20 mg/day. A ratio of RRR-alpha-tocopherol to grams of PUFA of approximately 0.4 has been suggested to insure health in adults. The daily recommended allowance of alpha-tocopherol has been set at 10 mg for men and 8 mg for women.

Epidemiological data is quite conflicting regarding the role of anti-oxidant supplementation in fighting off certain diseases. Some studies have suggested that low serum concentrations of antioxidants may be associated with an elevated risk of developing certain cancers. Four large randomized trials in the 1980's provided evidence. In a study conducted in China on approximately 30,000 men and women aged between 40 and 69 years of age, five years of supplementation with a combination of Vitamin E, Beta-carotene, and selenium reduced the rate of stomach cancer mortality by 21% and overall cancer mortality by 13%. A study on 540 patients with head and neck cancer being treated with radiation therapy, however, reported that Vitamin E administration, while capable of reducing side effects of the treatment, was associated with a higher cancer recurrence rate; differences did not reach significance though there was not the reduction in cancer recurrence that the investigators hoped for.

A review of 19 clinical trials involving Vitamin E use and 135,000 subjects concluded that individuals who took Vitamin E in doses greater than 400 IU increased their risk of dying by 4%; this study population also had a 13% greater risk of developing heart failure. Clearly, this data is hard to evaluate given the many variables involved and the unknown factor of just why the individuals were taking the high doses of Vitamin E in the first place, perhaps for an underlying illness that may have pre-disposed them to early death and heart disease.

There has been conflicting data regarding Vitamin E's role in preventing prostate cancer. One study reported a significant reduction in the incidence of prostate cancer in those who took alpha-tocopherol supplementation for a mean of 6 years. A study of more than 35,000 men taking Vitamin E, Selenium, or a combination of the two, however, failed to replicate these findings. Another study in male physicians evaluated the role of Vitamins E and C in the prevention of prostate and total cancer. This study also failed to demonstrate benefit from either of these supplements.

Vitamin K

Vitamin K consists of a group of compounds that contain a 2-methyl-1.4-naphthoquinone moiety. Compounds with Vitamin K activity are essential for the formation of prothrombin and at least five other proteins (factors VII, IX, and X and proteins C and S) that are necessary for the proper regulation of blood clotting. While Vitamin K is thought to also play a role in the biosynthesis of other proteins in the body, the only major finding associated with a deficiency is a defective coagulation of blood.

Vitamin K is absorbed in the intestine, primarily in the jejunum and ileum. Once again, normal biliary and pancreatic function appear to be necessary in order to achieve maximal absorption. Individuals who malabsorb fat are at high risk of developing a deficiency in Vitamin K.

Once absorbed, Vitamin K is transported via the lymph system in chylomicrons. It is initially concentrated in the liver and is then distributed among body tissues. Vitamin K makes its way into the cell membranes. The total body pool of Vitamin K is relatively small and its turnover is rapid. Liver stores of Vitamin K are found in two forms, approximately 10% being phylloquinone, derived from plants, and 90% menaquinones, thought to be synthesized by bacteria within the intestine. These latter products are not able to maintain adequate control of clotting on their own and thus we require additional dietary sources of Vitamin K.

In the liver, Vitamin K is necessary to form prothrombin, also known as coagulation factor II and factors VII, IX, X and proteins C and S. In the absence of Vitamin K, these proteins are still produced but remain non-functional. There are other Vitamin K dependent proteins in the bones, kidneys, and other tissues. These are thought to help bind calcium in the formation of bone and possibly help to synthesize some of the body's phospholipids, an essential component for cell integrity.

Vitamin K is plentiful in leafy green vegetables, providing 50 to 800 micrograms of Vitamin K per 100 gram portion. Smaller amounts of Vitamin K (1 to 50 micrograms/100 gram portion) are found in milk and other dairy products, meats, eggs, cereals, fruits and vegetables.

A normal American diet contains approximately 300 to 500 micrograms of Vitamin K. This amount will clearly vary depending on the intake of foods rich in Vitamin K. Normal prothrombin concentrations in the blood range from 80 to 120 micrograms per milliliter of blood and have been used to assess Vitamin K status as well as one measure of clotting time, the prothrombin time (PT). Dietary intake of Vitamin K should be approximately 1 microgram/kg body weight per day in order to maintain normal blood clotting. The RDA for Vitamin K has been set at approximately 80 micrograms per day for men and 63 micrograms for women. Chronic disease, medications, and poor diet are all risk factors for Vitamin K deficiency. Individuals taking antibiotics chronically are also at great risk due to their effect on eliminating intestinal bacteria essential for Vitamin K formation.

Even in large doses, Vitamin K appears to be non-toxic when taken orally. When menadione, a synthetic injectable form of Vitamin K is administered in toxic doses, however, hemolytic anemia and hyperbilirubinemia have been described and kernicterus has been reported in newborns.

Water-Soluble Vitamins

Vitamin C

Vitamin C, otherwise known as ascorbic acid, is a water-soluble vitamin with anti-oxidant properties. While some species are capable of producing ascorbic acid, man is dependent on dietary sources. Vitamin C is essential for proper formation of collagen from its components proline and lysine. It is also essential in the conversion of dopamine to norepinephrine and tryptophan to 5-hydroxytrytophan. It is also necessary in a number of chemical reactions in the body involving folic acid, histamine, tyrosine, corticosteroids, neuroendocrine peptides, and bile acids. Effects on white blood cells (leukocytes) and macrophages have been noted and Vitamin C has been implicated in a number of immune responses as well as helping in wound healing.

Vitamin C increases the absorption of iron from plant sources. Plasma concentrations of Vitamin C reach a plateau of 1.2 to 1.5 mg/dl at an intake of 90 to 150 mg/day with 80–90% of it being absorbed. Body stores of Vitamin C are approximately 3,000 mg in those who take 2,000 mg daily. At intakes of 60 to 100 mg per day, however, body stores are closer to 1,500 mg. Vitamin C is stored within the cells themselves and the concentration is several times that found in the blood. Excretion is mainly in the urine with oxalate, the major product formed at ingested doses of up to 100 mg/day. Higher intakes result in a greater elimination of ascorbic acid itself. At higher levels of ingestion, ascorbic acid is also degraded within the intestine to form carbon dioxide.

Vegetables and fruits contain relatively high concentrations of Vitamin C, especially green and red peppers, collard greens, broccoli, asparagus, spinach, tomatoes, strawberries, and citrus fruits. Vitamin C is present in small amounts in meat, fish, eggs, and dairy products; grains contain no Vitamin C. In recent years, there has been an increase in the daily intake of Vitamin C with the average intake currently in excess of 100 mg daily. This is supplemented by use of vitamins and additional use of ascorbic acid added to certain processed foods. The dietary allowance of Vitamin C is difficult to determine. As little as 10 mg per day prevents symptoms of deficiency (scurvy) and an intake of more than 200 mg per day results in it being excreted into the urine. Since Vitamin C must be taken regularly and is not well stored in the body, the RDA has been set at 60 mg per day. This amount is easily obtained in the American diet, though even here, individuals with specific food preferences may find themselves deficient in Vitamin C in the absence of supplemental sources such as a daily vitamin. Cigarette smokers have been described as having lower concentrations of ascorbic acid in the serum and white blood cells. This is thought to result not because of reduced intake of Vitamin C but rather an increase in its metabolism. For this reason, the intake of Vitamin C should be doubled in those who smoke regularly.

The classic deficiency state resulting from an inadequate intake of Vitamin C is the disease known as scurvy. This was a major problem in the past for those who were unable to obtain adequate quantities of foods rich in Vitamin C for prolonged periods of time such as sailors. This was a particularly difficult problem for the British navy who eventually solved their problem by providing all sailors with regular supplies of Vitamin C rich limes, thus the name "limies". Clinical findings associated with scurvy include swollen and bleeding gums, petechial hemorrhages, joint pain, and follicular hyperkeratosis. Once clinical disease is present, higher doses of Vitamin C high may be necessary to replete stores and reverse the disease process.

Vitamin C has been advocated as an antioxidant though there is conflicting data as to whether it offers any better protection than other available sources. Some studies have suggested that ascorbic acid may prevent the formation of carcinogenic nitrosamines by reducing nitrites. The ingestion of a diet rich in fruits and vegetables has been linked to lower rates of certain cancers. There is currently insufficient data, however, to conclude that Vitamin C is responsible for this reduction in cancer rates with more recent data unable to demonstrate an effect.

Vitamin C has also been implicated in reducing symptoms of viral illness associated with the common cold; there is insufficient evidence once again to prove that there is any benefit though several studies have demonstrated a somewhat shorter disease process in those individuals who took in excess of one gram of Vitamin C at the onset of "cold symptoms". Well controlled, double-blinded studies, however, have demonstrated only a minimal benefit or none at all. Vitamin C has been shown to reduce the onset of colds by 50% among people who engage in "extreme activities" such as marathon runners, skiers, and soldiers, all who are individuals exposed to significant cold or physical stress.

Vitamin C in large doses has also been implicated in reducing serum cholesterol levels, though this effect is not widely accepted as being large enough to have any clinical significance. While many persons take in excess of 1 gram of ascorbic acid daily without any apparent toxicity, the risk of calcium oxalate kidney stones remains a problem for at least some.

Vitamin C has recently received attention as having a possible protective effect against Alzheimer's disease when used in combination with high doses of Vitamin E. Combined use of Vitamins C and E in doses of at least 500 mg per day Vitamin C and greater than 400 IU per day of Vitamin E were studied as part of a large population-based investigation of the prevalence and incidence of Alzheimer's disease and other forms of dementia in Utah. Subjects aged 65 and older were assessed twice in 1996–1997 and again in 1998–2000. Over 3,000 individuals were asked about their use of any prescription or over-the-counter medication including supplemental vitamins. Approximately 17% of the subjects reported using Vitamin E or C supplements; these subjects tended to be younger, better educated, more commonly women, and in better general health as compared to those who reported no vitamin use. Twenty percent of the subjects used multivitamins that did not contain high doses of Vitamin C or E. There was a delay in onset of dementia among users of a combination of Vitamins C and E supplements even after correcting for the above variables found between the groups that used high doses of these vitamins and those who did not. They failed to observe any benefit from use of either vitamin alone or when taken in smaller doses. Additional studies are necessary prior to making any definite conclusion and once again, the potential for unwanted effects of Vitamins C and E must be considered.

Thiamine (Vitamin B1)

Thiamine is a necessary cofactor or coenzyme required for normal carbohydrate metabolism, an energy forming process in the body. It also plays a role in the metabolism of certain amino acids that are derived from protein sources and may also have a role in normal nerve membrane activity. With normal amounts taken in the diet, thiamin is absorbed in the proximal small intestine through a mechanism of active transport. Higher concentrations are absorbed passively as well; excess amounts are excreted into the urine in the form of thiamine acetic acid and other thiamine metabolites, including the pyrimidine and thiazolic forms. More than 20 metabolites of thiamine have been described in the urine.

Alcohol abuse and folate deficiency may lead to a malabsorption of thiamine. Caffeic acid and tannic acid found in coffee and tea act as thiamine antagonists in the body. Of note, individuals who have been severely malnourished and are re-fed may become deficient in thiamine as a result of thiamine's role in metabolizing ingested carbohydrates.

Thiamine deficiency affects carbohydrate metabolism and in the setting of a severe deficiency, the metabolic pathway is prevented from proceeding as normal. Prolonged deficiency of thiamine in the diet results in a disease entity referred to as beriberi. Primary symptoms include changes in the nervous and cardiovascular systems. Individuals who are affected may become confused, have a reduction in appetite, and complain of muscular weakness and an unsteady gait. They may also become paralyzed, have an inability to move the eyes normally, and may develop muscle wasting, a rapid heart beat, and have an enlarged heart that if not treated may lead to heart failure.

As stated previously, due to a complex metabolic process, the intake of glucose, either directly or as a result of carbohydrate ingestion, in the setting of a significant deficiency in thiamine may raise plasma levels of lactic and pyruvic acids. This may result in increased amounts of liver and heart muscle glycogen. This carbohydrate loading in the presence of thiamine deficiency may precipitate the classic nervous disorder known as Wernicke-Korsakoff syndrome. It may also increase peripheral accumulation of fluid, made even worse by exercise. Exercise leads to an accumulation of lactic and pyruvic acids; without a normal amount of thiamine, there is an inability to properly metabolize these products to form energy and they exert harmful effects on the body. Heart failure has been described in some, especially thiamine deficient children. Wernicke-Korsakoff syndrome is classically heralded by changes in mental status with short-term memory loss and "confabulation", or "making up stories", a classic finding.

While not a common deficiency, it is frequently observed in chronic alcoholics who have both reduced thiamine consumption and absorption and an increased requirement to metabolize products of ingested alcohol. Others more commonly affected include persons on chronic dialysis and individuals fed intravenously without attention to supplemental thiamine. Individuals who consume un-enriched white rice and white flour may also fail to obtain sufficient thiamine from natural sources. Thiamine is found in the "husk" of rice and wheat and thus thiamine deficiency has become more common as dietary preferences for "refined foods" developed over time. Individuals who consume large quantities of uncooked fish may also be deficient due to an enzyme, thiaminase, that is found in certain fish and is capable of breaking down thiamine.

Main dietary sources of thiamine include un-refined cereal grains, brewer's yeast, lean cuts of pork, organ meats, seeds, nuts and legumes. In the United States, grains and cereals are usually "enriched" with thiamine.

The recommended daily requirement of thiamine is 1.22 mg/day for men and 1.03 mg/day for women. Another way to look at this is by milligrams consumed per 1,000 kcal daily. Using this method, a thiamine allowance for adults has been set at 0.5 mg/1,000 kcal with a minimum of 1.0 mg/day recommended for those consuming less than 2,000 calories daily. Intake less than 0.2 mg/1,000 kcal in the diet appears to be the threshold below which deficiency states may develop though some argue that this critical level is closer to 0.5 mg/1,000 kcal in the diet. There is no data to suggest that thiamine requirements increase with age.

As with most other water-soluble vitamins, an excess oral intake of thiamine has not been shown to have toxic effects.

Riboflavin (Vitamin B2)

Riboflavin is a water-soluble vitamin that serves as a component of two flavin coenzymes-flavin mononucleotide (FMN) and flavin adenine dinucleotide (FAD). These serve to strengthen many energy forming reactions in the body and are involved in the conversion of tryptophan to niacin.

Riboflavin is absorbed in the proximal small intestine and is excreted in the urine. Good sources of riboflavin in the diet include animal protein sources such as meat, poultry, fish, and dairy products. Grains naturally contain relatively low levels. For this reason, producers add riboflavin in enriched and fortified grains and cereals. Green vegetables including broccoli, asparagus, spinach, and turnip greens contain relatively large amounts of riboflavin.

Intake less than 0.55 mg per day has been associated with clinical signs of riboflavin deficiency. It does take several months for deficiency states to develop in the absence of suitable dietary intake. The suggested minimum requirement has been set at 1.2 mg/day for most adults. While no cases of toxicity have been described from excessive intake of riboflavin orally, deficiency states are associated with oral lesions such as cheilosis and an inflammation at the angles of the mouth (angular stomatitis). Generalized seborrheic dermatitis, changes in the scrotal and vulval skin, and a normocytic anemia have also been described.

An adequate amount of riboflavin is essential to the normal functioning of both Vitamins B6 and niacin, and therefore a deficiency in riboflavin may have more profound effects than one might initially consider.

Niacin (Vitamin B3)

Niacin is a water-soluble vitamin that is largely derived from dietary sources of tryptophan. Niacin may be in the form of either nicotinic acid or nicotinamide, a component of two essential co-enzymes necessary for normal metabolism of fats and carbohydrates as well as for energy production, e.g. NAD and NADP. These co-enzymes are present in all cells.

A deficiency of niacin results in the serious disease of pellagra. Pellagra is characterized by changes in the skin (dermatitis), diarrhea, inflammation of the mucous membranes, and even dementia. Clinical disease appears to be worse after exposure to sunlight and is still found commonly in parts of Africa and Asia.

Niacin is found in relatively large quantities in meat. Milk and eggs also contain niacin though in smaller amounts. Fortunately, these foods also contain tryptophan and thus can provide a sufficient amount of precursor to insure an adequate niacin level. In general, protein rich foods contain approximately 1.0% tryptophan or in other words, 60 grams of protein provides 600 mg of tryptophan. More exactly, corn is 0.6% tryptophan by weight; other grains, fruits and vegetables, 1.0%; meat, 1.1%; milk, 1.4%; and eggs, 1.5%. Approximately 60 mg of tryptophan is equivalent to 1 mg of niacin, also referred to as a niacin equivalent or NE. While 25 to 40% of niacin comes from grain products in the diet, niacin is also added as part of the fortification process to grains. The average diet in the US supplies approximately 700 mg of tryptophan daily for women and 1,100 mg daily for men or between 27 and 40 mg of niacin, respectively.

The suggested daily requirement for niacin intake is 6.6 mg of niacin equivalents per 1,000 kcal intake. A diet consisting of less than 2,000 kcal should contain at least 13 mg of niacin equivalent from a combination of tryptophan and niacin.

Excessive intake of nicotinic acid, but not nicotinamide, may lead to vascular dilatation and flushing, common problems in persons taking nicotinic acid for therapeutic effects on reducing serum lipid levels. Very large doses have also been associated with a variety of side-effects including excessive loss of muscle glycogen and decreased removal of fatty acids from fat tissue during exercise. This may lead to weakness and reduced exercise tolerance.

Vitamin B6

Vitamin B6 consists in three forms, pyridoxine, pyridoxal, and pyridoxamine. They are converted as they pass through the liver, red blood cells and other tissues in the body to pyridoxal phosphate and pyridoxamine phosphate. These substances serve as co-enzymes necessary for normal protein, carbohydrate, and lipid metabolism. Absorbed through the intestine, Vitamin B6 must be taken in higher amounts as protein intake increases or a severe deficiency state may result. Vitamin B6 deficiency rarely occurs in isolation and is usually associated with other Vitamin B problems. Individuals who are deficient in B6 may present with dermatitis, anemia, and seizures.

Vitamin B6 is found in significant quantities in fish, chicken, pork, eggs and organ meats, especially liver and kidney. Unmilled rice, oats, soy beans, whole-wheat products, peanuts and walnuts are other good sources of Vitamin B6. It should be noted that freezing fruits and vegetables reportedly reduces B6 activity by as much as 15 to 70%; freezing cereals reduces activity by 50 to 90%; and meats by 50 to 70%. Freezing dairy products has little effect on B6 activity.

Numerous medications may reduce B6 by affecting its metabolism. Oral contraceptives have been associated with lower levels of B6.

The recommended daily allowance for Vitamin B6 is 2.0 mg per day for men and 1.6 mg per day for women. While this amount is felt to be suitable for individuals consuming up to 100 grams of protein a day for men and 60 mg per day for women, those consuming higher quantities may require higher Vitamin B6 intake. Fortunately, Vitamin B6 is usually found in high amounts in foods that are high sources of protein. Another way to calculate daily requirements is to use 0.016 mg Vitamin B6 per gram of protein consumed.

While not common, an excessively large intake of Vitamin B6 may result in ataxia, or unsteady gait, and a severe sensory neuropathy. This has been described with prolonged intakes of pyridoxine in excess of 100 mg daily. These symptoms resolve upon discontinuation of the excess amount though affected individuals may take months to fully recover.

Folate

Folate and folacin are compounds that have nutritional benefits similar to folic acid. These function as co-enzymes in the body and transport single carbon fragments necessary for normal amino acid and nucleic acid synthesis. Folate is widely distributed in foods with yeast, leafy vegetables, legumes and some fruits especially rich in content. Unfortunately, heat, oxidation and UV light may destroy folate's potency as may prolonged food storage, food preparation, and cooking. Approximately 90% of folate monoglutamate and 50 to 90% of folate polyglutamate is absorbed by the intestine.

The daily requirement of folate is approximately 50 micrograms; since not all folate in the diet is absorbed, most agree that 100 micrograms should be ingested daily. The RDA for folate has been set at 3 micrograms per kilogram body weight for men, non-pregnant, non-lactating women, and adolescents or a minimum of 200 micrograms for adult men and 180 micrograms for adult females. This quantity will not only ensure an adequate level of folate within the cells of the body but also provides sufficient amount for storage in the liver to protect against the development of a folate deficiency during periods of inadequate oral intake.

While high levels of folate ingestion in laboratory animals have been reported to cause kidney damage, there have been no reports of problems in humans even at doses of 10–15 milligrams daily for up to 4 months. Individuals on the anti-seizure medications phenytoin, phenobarbital, and primidone, however, are advised to avoid excessive doses of folate as they appear to compete for absorption in the intestine and brain and are capable of reducing the anti-seizure medication's effectiveness.

Folate deficiency may result in a megaloblastic anemia similar to that found in B12 deficiency. Neurological findings may also be noted including dementia and peripheral neuropathies, though not as frequently observed in B12 deficient individuals. The tongue may loose its normal architecture and become smooth and the intestine may also be affected due to an increase in the turnover of intestinal cells.

Folic acid supplementation has been associated in at least one study with a significant risk reduction for developing colon cancer. There remains conflicting data as to the effect folic acid supplementation may have on cardiovascular disease risk reduction with at least one well done study reporting a significant risk reduction, possibly related to its ability to reduce homocysteine levels that have been associated with inflammation.

Vitamin B12

Vitamin B12 is a generic term used to describe a variety of cobalamins that are necessary for metabolic processes throughout the body effecting lipid, carbohydrate and protein metabolism. Cyanocobalamin is the commercially available form of B12 used in vitamin preparations and is converted in the body to a usable form. Since methylcobalamin is essential in folate metabolism, folate and B12 interact and are necessary for the normal conversion of homocysteine to methionine, for protein biosynthesis, synthesis of purines and pyrimidines, for methylation reactions and for the maintenance of intracellular levels of folate.

B12 is absorbed in the ileum of the intestine but requires a substance known as gastric intrinsic factor. Intrinsic factor is a highly specific binding protein secreted by the parietal cells of the stomach. For this reason, anything that affects the ability of the body to produce intrinsic factor or affects the ileum may reduce B12 absorption.

Such problems may occur in persons with gastric atrophy as seen in aged individuals and the disease pernicious anemia that results from antibodies directed against the stomach's intrinsic factor producing parietal cells. This latter disease is also associated with achlorhydria or a reduction in acid production by the stomach. Individuals who have had a gastrectomy or who have had their pancreatic function impaired and thus a reduced production of enzymes necessary for the release of Vitamin B12 from binding proteins may also have a deficiency in Vitamin B12. In cases of Vitamin B12 deficiency, folate is unable to be converted to the form necessary for proper red cell production and thus a megaloblastic anemia may result.

Vitamin B12 is stored in the liver in quantities up to 10 mg. About 3 micrograms of B12 are secreted into the bile each day and largely re-absorbed in the ileum. Between 0.1 and 0.2% of Vitamin B12 is excreted each day and thus the RDA has been set at 2 micrograms per day for adults. Vitamin B12 is derived entirely from animal products including meat, fish, poultry, shellfish, eggs, milk, and dairy products. Since vegans do not consume adequate quantities of Vitamin B12 in their diet, supplements are essential to ensuring good health. Vitamin B12 is quite stable during food preparation.

Deficiency states of Vitamin B12 are quite common, especially in the elderly who have the highest rate of pernicious anemia. B12 deficiency, however, may also result from lack of intake of B12 containing foods for prolonged periods of time, intestinal tape worms that compete for the B12 itself, and individuals with "blind loop" syndromes from prior intestinal surgery that leads to bacterial overgrowth and increased breakdown of B12 prior to it being able to be absorbed. Common findings associated with deficiency include a sore tongue, paresthesias, or numbness and tingling of the legs, weakness, and dementia. A megaloblastic or macrocytic anemia is characteristic, though not essential to the diagnosis, and is associated with classic hyper-segmented polymorphonuclear neutrophils. Since this may also be seen in persons deficient in folate, it is necessary that both vitamins be assessed early as folate replacement may correct the blood abnormality but not the neurological findings.

Large doses of B12 have not been associated with harmful effects and in fact, it has long been used as a "tonic" in medical practice. There has been no proven benefit when given to individuals with normal levels of Vitamin B12 other than unsubstantiated reports of feelings of "renewed strength and vigor" on a case-by-case basis. This more likely results from its ruby red color and the "power of suggestion" than any scientific reason.

Individuals with deficiency states may be treated with oral supplements of 1 microgram per day as long as there is no problem with B12 absorption. If there is, 100 micrograms can be given as a monthly injection. While some still advocate for a multi-staged Schilling Test to best determine the exact reason for the B12 deficiency — whether it is from inadequate intake, absorption, or increased break-down — others argue it is more cost-effective, particularly in older persons, to conduct an accurate history of intake and medication use and then treat with supplemental B12 on a regular basis if no obvious cause is found.

Biotin

Biotin is essential for proper handling of carbon dioxide in the body and for the production of glucose and fatty acids essential for energy production. While fruit and meat are poor sources of biotin, liver, egg yolks, soy flour, cereals and yeast are rich in biotin content. Unfortunately, biotin present in wheat is not able to be utilized. Biotin is also produced by microorganisms found in the intestine. Little is known regarding specific requirements for biotin in the diet. A daily dose of 60 micrograms has been used to maintain health in individuals without normal intestinal function.

Biotin deficiency, although rare, is associated with anorexia, nausea, vomiting, glossitis, depression, alopecia or hair loss, and dry scaly skin. There may also be an increase in bile pigments and serum cholesterol. No reports of toxicity have been described.

Pantothenic Acid

Pantothenic acid is a B-complex vitamin that serves as a co-enzyme necessary for proper fatty acid synthesis and degradation, energy production from carbohydrates, and synthesis of steroid hormones, porphyrins, and acetylcholine. Porphyrins play an important role in the structure of hemoglobin, the main ingredient of our red blood cells; acetylcholine is an essential mediator for proper nerve action and memory.

Pantothenic acid is found in large quantities in a variety of foods including meats, whole grains, and legumes. Smaller amounts are found in milk, fruit and vegetables. The intestinal flora is thought to produce this vitamin as well and may be responsible for the lack of a deficiency state even in the absence of dietary intake. There have been several case reports of an unusual presentation of "burning feet" that responds to pantothenic supplementation described in severely malnourished individuals. The usual dietary intake of pantothenic acid in the US is between 5 and 10 mg per day.

CHAPTER
8

The Role of Minerals
in Successful Aging

Calcium

An adequate intake of calcium is essential for our bones to remain healthy throughout life. While found in almost all cells in the body and essential for proper function of the heart, muscles, and nervous system, 99% of our calcium is found in the bones. Every year approximately 30% of our bone structure is new as a result of continuous "re-modeling". In order that we keep in "balance" and continue to replace the bone mass that is lost, we must have sufficient calcium intake as well as normal hormonal balance. While our bone mass peaks between ages 21 and 24, there is a great deal of variation in bone density based on a variety of factors. Just how strong our bones remain throughout our lives, however, is mostly within our control. Osteoporosis is a disease that affects millions of Americans and is *not* an inevitable consequence of growing old as previously thought!

Bone health represents only one aspect of calcium's importance in the body as the mineral is also necessary for the formation and maintenance of healthy teeth and plays a key role in the blood clotting process. It also is essential for proper nerve, heart and muscle functioning.

Many factors help determine our bone strength including our genetic predisposition for developing osteoporosis. Osteoporosis is more common in individuals who have family members with a history of osteoporosis and in women from Northern European and Asian descent. Proper bone health can be negatively affected by many factors including intake of caffeine, alcohol, and colas; weight less than 127 pounds; multiple births; Vitamin D status; medications including steroid use and certain medications used to treat asthma;

post-menopausal status; diseases such as hyperthyroidism; and regular maintenance of physical activity.

Approximately 25 to 50% of calcium in the diet is absorbed in the intestine using an active transport process. Vitamin D in the form of 1,25 dihydroxycholecalciferol is necessary for this active calcium transport that utilizes a calcium-binding protein in the intestine. Passive absorption may also occur. High oxalate and phytate in the diet may reduce the ability to absorb calcium. Additionally, unabsorbed fatty acids as may result from diseases of the intestine, may bind calcium and also reduce absorption.

Calcium balance is largely controlled by parathyroid hormone, calcitonin and Vitamin D. Vitamin D stimulates intestinal absorption of calcium and reduces excretion through the kidney. High sodium and protein intake is associated with reduced calcium absorption and a higher requirement in the diet. Unfortunately, adequate intake of calcium is rare in the typical US diet with studies demonstrating as many as 50% of persons failing to meet daily requirements.

While the range of recommended calcium intake has been set between 800 and 1,500 mg per day, this requirement varies greatly depending on one's age, sex, health and bone status. Women who are pregnant or breast-feeding require higher intakes of calcium due to the increased demand that these physiological states place on bones. After age 60, one's ability to absorb dietary calcium reportedly declines, thus increasing the amount required to between 1,200 and 1,500 mg daily. Once osteoporosis has been detected, a daily intake of 1,500 mg of calcium is recommended.

Vitamin D must also be maintained within a certain range and may require supplements to insure that a proper level is being achieved. Vitamin D is produced through a series of chemical reactions that convert cholesterol in the skin with the help of ultra-violet light to a compound known as D3. This substance circulates throughout the body and when it passes through the liver, undergoes a conversion to form 25 Hydroxy (OH)-D3, a substance that is 1.5 times more potent than D3 itself. To make this even more potent, mother nature adds another hydroxy (OH) group onto circulating 25OH-D3 when it passes through the kidney to form 1,25 di-OH D3, and by doing this makes a substance that is approximately 5 times more potent than the original Vitamin D. It is easy to see that anything that may interfere with any aspect of this process can lead to a deficiency in Vitamin D. In addition, Vitamin D is a fat-soluble vitamin and anything that causes fats to be malabsorbed will also cause a deficiency. Pure Vitamin D deficiency results in the disease known as rickets in children and osteomalacia in adults. This is also associated with an increased risk of fractures. While a certain amount of Vitamin D is essential to proper bone health, too much may result in hypervitaminosis D, or Vitamin D toxicity. This may result in excessively high levels of calcium in the blood and can be fatal if untreated. Proper supervision is essential.

The best source of calcium is dairy products with approximately 300 mg of elemental calcium in 8 ounces of milk. Skim milk contains the same amount of calcium as whole milk. Yogurt contains an equivalent quantity, though few people realize that the average size of a commercially available container for a single serving of yogurt is rarely 8 ounces in size, but rather 4 or 6. One ounce of natural cheese and 2 ounces of processed cheese also contains an equivalent amount of calcium, though ice cream and cottage cheese vary depending on the content of air, fruit, and other supplements that are added. Cream cheese should not be considered a cheese as it contains almost no calcium. While other foods contain variable amounts of calcium, it is exceedingly difficult to obtain sufficient calcium in the absence of dairy products in the diet. Foods with approximately 100 mg of calcium per serving include salmon with bones, collards, turnip greens, instant farina and kale. Sardines with bones are a relatively good source of calcium with 2.25 ounces containing the calcium found in 8 ounces of milk. Unfortunately, it would take 10 Eggs, 29 tablespoons of peanut butter, 7.75 pounds of tuna, 14 cups of rice, and 13 cups of oatmeal to give you that equivalent quantity of calcium.

Due to the large reservoir of calcium in the body, hypocalcemia is an extremely rare condition in persons who fail to consume adequate amounts of calcium. Calcium deficiency may result from inadequate circulating levels of parathyroid hormone and Vitamin D or from the use of chelating agents. Hypocalcemia may present with numbness and tingling due to neuromuscular excitability, muscle cramping, tetany and even convulsions. Electrocardiographic findings include a prolonged Q-T interval.

The most common clinical finding associated with long term calcium imbalance is osteoporosis. The World Health Association defines someone as having osteoporosis if they have a bone density more than 2.5 standard deviations below a standard reference in the absence of other identifiable causes. Individuals who fall below 1.0 standard deviation from the standard reference have what is referred to as osteopenia. This latter term refers to a "thinning" of the bone mass and is a precursor to osteoporosis, or "porous bone". In this latter case, the support structure of bone is so weak that one's own weight may result in the bone breaking. Clearly, anything that provides additional stress such as a fall or heavy weight can lead to an increased risk of fracture. While hip fractures are common with over 250,000 every year in the US alone, compression fractures of the spine often go unrecognized and over time lead to a significant curvature of the spine (kyphosis) and a reduction in height, bone pain, and even compromised lung function. Fortunately, osteoporosis and its harmful sequellae may be avoided with life-long attention to prevention.

Iodine

Iodine is a trace element that is essential to the formation of our thyroid hormones. Thyroid hormones are a major determinant of our metabolism and are produced through a series of enzymatic processes in the thyroid gland, an H-shaped gland located in the neck lying over our trachea. Iodine is "trapped" by the thyroid gland and undergoes a series of conversions starting with mono-iodo-thyronine. As iodine is added to this compound, di-iodothyronine, tri-iodothyronine, and tetra-iodothyronine are formed, named after the number of iodines that have been added. It is the compound, 3,5,3',5' tetra-iodothyronine that is commonly known as T4 or thyroxine. It is this product that circulates in the body and once again through a series of enzymatic degradations forms 3,5,3' tri-iodothyronine, T3, a more potent form of thyroid hormone. Approximately 80% of T3 is formed from the removal of one iodine from T4 as it circulates through the liver, kidney and muscle. The rest of T3 is made by the thyroid gland itself. As we age and the thyroid has a harder time keeping up with thyroid hormone production, the thyroid itself makes a greater amount of T3; this substance is 3–5 times more metabolically active than T4 and requires one less iodine to produce. The body has a "check and balance" system to help maintain metabolic equilibrium that involves not only the thyroid gland but also the pituitary gland and the hypothalamus, a portion of our brains.

Thyroid hormone exerts most of its metabolic effect through the control of protein synthesis. Receptors for thyroid hormone have been identified within the cell nucleus, cell membrane and mitochondria. Proper amounts of thyroid hormone are essential for normal metabolism, caloric expenditure, and mental and physical well being.

Iodine is absorbed from the diet and circulates largely as organic iodine, though approximately 5% is in the form of iodide. Most of the organic iodine is in thyroid hormone. The daily iodine requirement for adults is approximately 1 to 2 micrograms/kg body weight. Ocean born seafoods and seaweed have high concentrations of iodine. Dairy products and eggs have variable iodine contents depending on the iodine placed in the animal feed. Vegetables are low in iodine content with amounts varying with the iodine content in the soil they are grown in. In recent years, iodine has been added to bread and salt. Current levels of iodine supplement provide 76 micrograms of iodine per gram of salt, but only if one consumes "iodized salt". There is still salt being sold without supplemental iodine so the consumer must know what type of salt they are buying and why it is important to take one form or the other.

Iodine deficiency may have significant consequences. The body strives to maintain a normal balance of thyroid hormone. The first response to a low intake of iodine is an increase in the body's level of serum TSH, produced in the pituitary as a regulatory hormone. This leads over time to an increase in the size of the thyroid gland, or goiter, in an attempt to "trap" iodine more efficiently. There is also a greater shift by the thyroid to produce T3, a hormone that is 3 to 5 times more potent than T4 and requires one less iodine, similar to what happens as part of the aging process but for different reasons. If these responses still fail to produce sufficient amounts of thyroid hormone, a hypothyroid state will result.

Children with inadequate amounts of thyroid early in life will have stunted growth, mental retardation, and other systemic changes. Adults will have symptoms of hypothyroidism, including fluid retention, lethargy, coarse hair and skin, constipation, slowed heart rate, among other potentially life-threatening findings.

While a deficiency of iodine produces hypothyroidism, a high intake may also lead to goiter formation due to iodine's effect on blocking thyroid hormone production, a process known as organification, when plasma iodine concentrations exceed 15–25 micrograms/ml. A daily intake of between 50 and 1,000 micrograms per day is considered to be safe and adequate for normal health. Excess amounts of iodine consumed may lead to hyperthyroidism in persons who have underlying abnormalities of thyroid hormone production, such as persons with enzymatic defects, or in those who come from areas of iodine deficiency. The thyroid gland has already compensated to these situations by altering the way thyroid hormone is produced, either making the more active form of thyroid hormone or being more efficient in thyroid hormone's production; in this case the additional iodine adds "fuel to the fire". Fortunately, the hyperthyroidism that results from this is transient.

Iron

Iron is an essential nutrient and a component of life sustaining hemoglobin, the oxygen carrying molecule within our red blood cells. It is also one of the building blocks of myoglobin and a number of enzymes. Approximately 30% of the body's iron is stored in the spleen, liver, and bone marrow in the form of ferritin and hemosiderin and a small amount circulates on the transport protein, transferrin.

Iron is absorbed by the intestinal mucosa. Heme and non-heme forms of iron are absorbed by different mechanisms. Heme iron is readily absorbable and constitutes approximately 40% of the total iron in animal tissues. The remaining 60% of the iron in animal tissues and all of the iron in vegetables is in a non-heme form. Non-heme iron absorption is increased by organic acids, such as ascorbic acid. Substances such as calcium phosphate, phytates, bran, polyphenols such as those in tea, and antacids may decrease non-heme iron absorption. In other words, iron in the diet is largely in the form of ferrous iron and is converted to the ferric form in the stomach under acidic conditions. Without this transformation, only 1% of dietary iron is absorbed. The percentage of iron absorbed in the diet decreases as the amount of iron present increases. Absorption of iron also depends on the iron status of the individual. Mean absorption of dietary iron is relatively low when body stores are high but increase when stores drop. This is nature's way of maintaining adequate iron stores under normal circumstances, storing what is required for reserves, and avoiding excessive quantities that may lead to toxic states.

As we age, we have a reduced amount of acid production by the parietal cells of the stomach. Although few develop a complete inability to produce acid, or achlorohyria, those with diseases such as pernicious anemia or who take anti-acid medications or acid production inhibitors may have a reduced ability to absorb iron through the diet. Since stores of iron in the body remain for long periods of time, this in itself rarely produces problems. When coupled with blood loss as may occur during times of menstruation or bleeding from the GI tract, however, a deficiency in iron may result. Even if there are sufficient stores of iron in the body, some individuals with chronic illness are unable to utilize this iron to produce normal red blood cells. This latter phenomenon leads to an entity known as an "anemia of chronic disease".

True iron deficiency results in microcytosis or small red blood cells and anemia. If anemia is defined as values which are more than two standard deviations below the mean, then a hemoglobin value of <13.5 g/dL and <12.0 g/dL for men and women, respectively represents anemia.

The most significant clinical finding associated with anemia is a reduction in physical endurance with most persons complaining of fatigue. Iron deficiency has also been associated with a reduction in immune function though no data exists demonstrating an actual effect on infection fighting ability. In children, iron deficiency has been associated with apathy, short attention span, reduced learning ability, and irritability. Blood loss is the most common cause of an iron deficiency; anemia may be due to other causes and thus an evaluation as to the cause of the anemia is necessary prior to blaming it on any one cause.

Iron is readily available in the diet with meat, fish, eggs, vegetables and fortified cereals our major sources. It has been estimated that women have an average iron store of approximately 300 mg and men, 1,000 mg. This is thought to provide sufficient reserve against periods of negative iron balance and in the absence of blood loss, should be adequate for several months even if no additional iron was consumed. Men loose an average of 1 mg of iron per day in the absence of excess blood loss.

Women average an additional 0.5 mg iron loss per day during their active menstrual periods, though this amount varies greatly from woman to woman and may be as high as an additional 1.5 mg per day on average. It is for this reason that many more women are anemic than men during their reproductive years. Based on normal amounts of absorption, the daily requirement of iron necessary to maintain proper health has been estimated at 10 mg for men and 15 mg for menstruating women per day. Post-menopausal women have the same daily requirement of iron as men, e.g. 10 mg per day.

Iron toxicity rarely occurs from excess intake of dietary sources of iron in the absence of a genetic pre-disposition to excess iron absorption and deposition. This disorder, known as hemochromatosis, may be present in as many as 4% of the population and is caused by an autosomal recessive gene. Some studies have reported as high as a 14% prevalence rate of individuals with a carrier state. If affected, toxic levels of iron accumulate in the heart, pancreas, testes, among other organs and may lead to life-threatening consequences. While not universally accepted, excess intake of iron may be associated with a higher rate of cardiac disease and thus caution is advised to avoid excessive intake as may occur from medicinal supplements. This is particularly true for men and post-menopausal women who are no longer menstruating.

Zinc

Zinc is an essential component of certain enzymes in the body that help to regulate cell division, growth, wound healing, and proper functioning of the immune system. It also appears to play a role in our sense of smell and taste. As with iron, requirements vary depending on the individual's zinc status; relatively large amounts of zinc are stored in bone and muscle. Despite this, there is a short half-life of zinc in the body. One's diet largely determines the availability of zinc. Interactions with other dietary components, such as protein, phytates, fiber, and some minerals influence our ability to absorb zinc; higher amounts are absorbed in association with the intake of milk, soy products, meat, and certain grains.

Individuals who are deficient in zinc may report a loss of appetite and a decline in taste. There may also be growth retardation, changes in the skin, and even immunological abnormalities. Zinc deficiency during pregnancy may lead to developmental disorders in off-spring and men with severe deficiency may have hypogonadism, low levels of testosterone, and infertility. Problems with wound healing have also been described in persons with zinc deficiency.

Approximately 70% of zinc in the diet is derived from animal products such as meat, eggs, and seafoods, particularly oysters. Most of the zinc consumed from other foods comes from cereals though it is also found in brewer's yeast, milk, beans, and wheat germ. It has been reported that increasing dietary intake of phosphorous increases zinc requirements due to a reduction in zinc absorption. The average American diet provides between 10 and 15 mg of zinc per day, though more recent data suggest somewhat lower amounts in the older person's diet. The minimal requirement for daily zinc intake has been set at 15 mg and 12 mg for men and women, respectively.

While not common, excess intake of zinc may impair proper copper status in the body, interfere with iron absorption, lead to impaired formation of red blood cells, neutropenia, and problems with immune system functioning. A reduction in high density lipoprotein (HDL) cholesterol, the good form of cholesterol, has also been described in individuals who consume high amounts of zinc for prolonged periods of time. For these reasons, chronic ingestion of zinc supplements in excess of 10–15 mg per day is strongly discouraged.

It is important to insure an adequate intake of zinc, though caution is advised not to take mega-doses that may provide a potentially harmful excess. The full potential benefit of zinc in the diet still remains in need of more scientific study. Although the prostate gland normally contains a high concentration of zinc and a deficiency of zinc has been linked to lower levels of testosterone, there is no scientific data to suggest that taking zinc improves potency or has any effect on improving prostate health. Oysters, rich in zinc, have long had a reputation for being able to promote potency but no causal relationship, has ever been found. Zinc has also been reported to protect against age-related macular-degeneration, the leading cause of blindness in the elderly that is thought to result from oxidative damage from free radicals. Additional studies need to be done to better define the role of zinc in this disease process. Zinc has even been touted as useful in fighting the common cold. To date, several studies have reported that the use of zinc in the form of a lozenge may reduce the duration of a cold by as much as three days. These studies have not withstood the scientific rigor necessary to make a definite conclusion and many studies have failed to prove any benefit.

For now, zinc supplements are not recommended other than in a dose found in a daily vitamin that provides the minimum daily requirement. If you are taking high doses of calcium and/or are a vegan, however, a simple multi-vitamin and mineral supplement with zinc is suggested. Once again, there is nothing to suggest that a higher dose of zinc should be taken and some evidence to suggest that it should be avoided.

Selenium

Selenium plays an essential role in maintaining an adequate defense against toxic oxidants. It is an essential component of the enzyme glutathione peroxidase. While still controversial, Chinese scientists in 1979 reported an association between low selenium levels and a form of cardiomyopathy, a problem with heart muscle function, effecting children and young women. Although animal studies have demonstrated problems resulting from selenium deficiency, few findings have been observed in humans. Muscular discomfort and weakness have both been reported in a limited number of individuals being fed entirely by intravenous methods using a selenium deficient diet; selenium supplementation corrected these symptoms. A form of cardiomyopathy was also described in these patients.

Selenium has been suggested as a potent anti-oxidant that may have beneficial effects in preventing degenerative diseases and certain forms of cancer. Most of these claims are based on animal studies and no data regarding selenium's preventive effects on human cancer is currently available to support this claim. One well designed study that provided men with large doses of selenium and Vitamin E, either alone or in combination, failed to demonstrate any difference in the incidence of prostate cancer.

Selenium is found in bountiful amounts in seafood, and kidney and liver organs. Other meats and fish contain less selenium; grain and seeds vary in content depending on the soil in which they grow. Fruits and vegetables contain little selenium. The usual diet contains approximately 100 micrograms of selenium per day with the suggested minimum requirement set at 70 and 55 micrograms per day for men and women, respectively.

Excessive intake of selenium in excess of 1 mg per day may lead to symptoms of nausea, abdominal pain, diarrhea, hair and nail changes, peripheral neuropathy, fatigue, and irritability. An increased incidence of diabetes mellitus has also been suggested in at least one study administering a supra-physiological dose of selenium.

Copper

Copper is an essential nutrient that is utilized in the body by certain proteins and enzymes, some of which are essential for the proper utilization of iron. Although rare, copper deficiency in animal models has been associated with anemia, skeletal defects, demyelination and degeneration of the nervous system, reproductive failure, myocardial degeneration, and decreased arterial elasticity. Low levels of copper may result from inadequate amounts in the diet or disease states that result in low proteins and thus an inability to provide adequate amounts of the protein that carries copper, ceruloplasmin. In severe cases of deficiency, anemia, neutropenia, and severe bone de-mineralization have been described in copper deficient children and growth retardation has also been reported. Epidemiological and experimental studies in animals suggest a positive correlation between the zinc-to-copper ratio in the diet and the incidence of cardiovascular disease. Individuals consuming low amounts of copper in the diet have also been found to have higher levels of cholesterol, glucose intolerance, and heart related abnormalities.

Copper is found in a variety of foods with particularly high amounts found in liver, seafood, nuts, and seeds. Most diets in the U.S. provide a daily intake of approximately 1.0 to 3.0 mg. A minimum intake of between 1.5 and 3.0 mg per day is recommended. To date, no abnormalities have been described in persons taking up to 10 mg daily.

Manganese

Manganese is essential for the proper functioning of certain enzymes in the body including decarboxylases, hydrolases, kinases and transferases. While rare, deficiencies have been associated with growth retardation, congenital abnormalities, abnormal formation of bone and cartilage, and impaired glucose tolerance. Fortunately, manganese is abundant in whole grains and cereal products and is also present in vegetables and fruits. Tea has also been found to be rich in manganese. The minimum daily requirement is 2.0 to 5.0 mg per day. Toxicity rarely occurs other than from occupational exposure to toxic levels in which case neurotoxicity may result. Although not recommended, an occasional intake of up to 10 mg per day is considered to be safe.

Fluoride

Fluorine (frequently named after its ionic form, fluoride) is present in small amounts in almost all soils, water, plants and animals and is incorporated into bones and tooth enamel in proportion to intake. While fluorine is not considered an essential element, it has been shown to have a valuable effect on maintaining proper dental health as its introduction as a supplement to water supplies in many communities has had a direct effect on reducing cavity formation and preserving dentition. The benefit on bone health is much more controversial with studies demonstrating a higher bone density in people residing in communities with high-fluoride content in their drinking water (4 to 5.8 mg/liter) as compared to those with less or no fluoride present. Of note, higher fluoride levels may lead to more dense but in fact more brittle bone with an actual increased rate of bone fracture. Excess fluorine intake may result in a chronic condition known as fluorosis and may also affect muscle, kidney, and nerve functioning. While some have even argued that fluorine intake may predispose to a higher rate of cancer, the data does not support this claim. The estimated range for a safe intake of fluoride for adults is 1.5 to 4.0 mg per day derived from all sources. Younger aged individuals should not have more than 2.5 mg per day; intakes of 0.1 to 1 mg are recommended during the first year of life and 0.5 to 1.5 mg per day for children up to age 3. Higher amounts have been associated with "mottled teeth" and are to be avoided.

Free fluoride as it exists in water is more readily available for use by the body than the protein-bound fluorine found in certain foods. Approximately 65% of sodium fluoride, used as a supplement to drinking water in certain communities, some milk products and baby formulas, is absorbed. The Food and Nutrition Board recommends fluoridation of public water supplies if natural fluoride levels are below 0.7 mg per liter.

Chromium

Chromium is necessary for normal glucose metabolism as it acts as a cofactor for insulin action. Impaired glucose tolerance and even a diabetes-like syndrome have both been described in chromium deficient animals. Chromium concentrations decline with age in most tissues, though concentrations in the lung reportedly increase. Intestinal absorption of chromium is in proportion to the total amount present with 0.5% absorbed when the daily intake is 40 micrograms or higher; approximately 2% is absorbed when lower amounts are in the diet. Of note, impaired glucose tolerance and even coronary artery disease have been associated with low concentrations of chromium found in blood and hair.

The recommended daily intake of chromium is between 50 and 200 micrograms daily. While bronchial cancer has been associated with toxic exposure to chromium chronically in an occupational setting, few if any side effects have been described from dietary intake in excess of recommended levels.

Molybdenum

Molybdenum is a necessary component of several enzymes including xanthine oxidase, aldehyde oxidase, and sulfite oxidase. Animal studies using goats have suggested that deficiencies may lead to anorexia, impaired ability to reproduce, and a shortened life expectancy. Human data regarding molybdenum deficiency is extremely sparse with rare reports of irritability, amino acid intolerance, and even coma found in the literature.

Foods rich in molybdenum include milk, beans, breads and cereals. The recommended minimum requirement for molybdenum has been set at between 75 and 250 micrograms daily for adults. Intakes in excess of 10 mg per day reportedly may lead to gout-like symptoms with elevated blood levels of molybdenum, uric acid and xanthine oxidase. An increased loss of copper in the urine has also been described.

9

The Role of Fiber
in Successful Aging

Fiber is essential for normal bowel mobility and function. In addition, fiber has been increasingly recognized as a natural way to improve blood sugar and even cholesterol. In modern times, our diets have become more "refined" and our fiber intake greatly reduced. The average intake of fiber in America is approximately 12 grams daily, less than half of what it should be for optimal health. Studies have demonstrated that societies that consume 30 or more grams of fiber a day have less colon cancer, constipation, diverticulosis, gallbladder disease, hypercholesterolemia, and hemorrhoids. In general, one third of one's daily fiber intake should be in the form of a soluble fiber and two thirds as insoluble fiber. Unfortunately, few Americans consume adequate quantities of any form of fiber. Studies that have reported "little benefit" from fiber intake have based their conclusions on groups of individuals consuming lower levels than may be necessary, though more typical of the usual American diet culture. Depending on what outcome is being measured, there may also be an inappropriate conclusion made regarding fiber's benefit or lack of it.

Many persons have given up the idea of increasing fiber in their diet due to bad initial experiences — increasing the quantity of fiber in one's diet too quickly may result in abdominal cramping, indigestion, bloating and gas! A scheduled plan to increase fiber in the diet is the best way to achieve one's individual goal. For some, dietary supplements may be the only way to achieve this high amount of fiber intake; others may be able to more easily incorporate fiber rich foods into their daily diets.

It is essential that we become familiar regarding foods that are good sources of both soluble and insoluble fiber and learn how to incorporate these into our everyday diets. Foods particularly rich in fiber include apples, barley, beans, legumes, fruits and vegetables, oatmeal, oat bran and brown rice. High fiber foods are digested more slowly so they do not cause spikes in blood sugar levels and rapid swings in insulin levels such as one may experience following intake of potatoes, bread and sweets. Water-soluble fibers include pectin, gums, mucilages, algal polysaccharides, some hemicelluloses, and some storage polysaccharides. These appear to have a greater effect on lowering serum cholesterol as compared to water-insoluble fibers. Oat bran, a rich source of soluble fiber, has been identified as particularly helpful in reducing cholesterol levels. Soluble fibers appear to increase fecal elimination of bile acids and cholesterol and thus stimulate hepatic uptake of LDL-cholesterol. Serum total cholesterol may decrease 0.5 to 2% per gram of soluble fiber and lower serum total cholesterol by approximately 15%. Simple changes to the diet can make a BIG difference. For example, every 8 ounce cup of whole wheat flour contains 15 grams of fiber as compared to only 4 grams in the same amount of white flour.

Guar and pectin have also been identified as a way to help keep blood sugar within better control and reducing the harmful swings that often lead to high insulin levels. Clearly, not all fiber is created equal and this too must be individually tailored to one's specific goals and needs. Another particular benefit from fiber is the "full feeling" it provides, an excellent adjunct to any weight reduction program.

The following are some comparative data from the US Department of Agriculture Database regarding fiber content in common foods.

Food	Serving Size	Fiber Content (grams)
Prunes	1 cup	16.4
Peas	1 cup	16.3
Black beans	1 cup	15.0
Pinto beans	1 cup	14.7
Oat bran	1 cup	14.5
Kidney beans (red)	1 cup	13.1
Lima beans	1 cup	10.8
Soybeans	1 cup	10.3
Pear, Asian	1 pear	9.9
Raspberries	1 cup	8.4

CHAPTER

10

Fat, Cholesterol and Illness

The American diet all too frequently contains an excessive amount of fat, especially saturated fat. While most agree that no more than 30% of calories should be derived from fats in the diet, the average American obtains closer to 40% of their calories from fat each day. Those on a low carbohydrate diet obtain calories mostly from protein and fat, and are at even greater risk of exceeding recommended allowances. A certain amount of fat is necessary for proper health and for the maintenance of our nervous system. It also provides 9 calories per gram and thus is an excellent source of calories for those who require them as compared to the 4 calories per gram that we get from foods rich in protein and carbohydrate. Fat is an excellent source of calories if necessary with 99% being utilized by the body. Eskimos have consumed high fat diets for generations as a way of obtaining the necessary calories to maintain their body temperature and provide necessary excess calories that could be converted to fat to insulate them from the cold environment. This survival tool, however, is not a benefit to the majority of individuals on this planet and limiting fat content in the diet to no more than 30% of total calories consumed is strongly advised with an emphasis placed on monounsaturated fats.

Fat comes in several forms and may be saturated, monounsaturated, or polyunsaturated. This nomenclature relates to the number of hydrogen bonds that connect the carbon atoms that make up the fat. Certain fats are naturally saturated, such as fats derived from animals and certain vegetables such as palm and coconut. Other fats can be "saturated" as part of the production process as occurs when liquid oils are converted into semi-solid form, such as is the case with margarine. Here a polyunsaturated fat in liquid form such as from corn or safflower is made into a partially saturated or "hydrogenated" fat. These are also referred to as "trans-fats" and have been implicated in promoting heart disease. Most agree that less than 10% of calories should come from saturated fat in any form; saturated fat has most commonly been associated with a greater risk of cardiovascular disease. The remaining fats can be derived from polyunsaturated or monounsaturated fats, with the latter of these two now considered to be the most beneficial and "heart healthy".

A Mediterranean diet high in vegetables, fruits, and cereal grains and low in meat has been shown capable of reducing both heart disease and the risk of developing diabetes. Several studies have shown that virgin olive oil used in moderation may protect against insulin resistance and the metabolic syndrome (obesity, lipid abnormalities, insulin resistance, and hypertension) that is associated with heart disease. The Mediterranean diet has also been associated with lower plasma concentrations of inflammatory markers and markers of endothelial dysfunction. While the main fat in this diet comes from olive oil, an oil rich in monounsaturated fats, canola oil has also been shown to have similar benefit if used in equal quantities. Unfortunately, many persons upon hearing that olive oil or canola oil is "cardiac protective" choose to incorporate these into their diets without regard to the quantity being used. Benefit is based on a similar amount being used as compared to other oils and not if used in greater quantity. Many people are under the assumption that canola oil is corn based. This is not the case; canola oil is derived from the rape seed.

Fats from dietary sources consist of a mixture of lipids that are mostly triglycerides. They also contain various amounts of cholesterol, phytosterols, glycolipids, sphingolipids, and phospholipids. In addition to being a major source of energy, fats in the diet furnish essential fatty acids, serve as a carrier for fat-soluble vitamins, and provide food with flavor and consistency. Almost all ingested fat, whether it comes from animal or vegetable sources, is absorbed by the body and able to be utilized. Less than 5% of ingested fats remain unabsorbed and are excreted in the feces. Short-chain triglycerides can be absorbed directly through the intestine while long-chain triglycerides must first be acted upon by digestive juices from the pancreas, pancreatic lipase, and bile salts.

There are three essential fatty acids, linoleic acid, linolenic acid and arachidonic acid. These fatty acids serve as precursors to substances that are essential for health including the prostaglandins, thromboxanes, prostacyclins, and leukotrienes. Alpha-linolenic acid, referred to as ALA, is converted to an omega-3 fatty acid and is essential for the normal functioning of the central nervous system, brain, and cell membranes throughout the body. They may also provide protection against heart disease. ALA is found in plentiful amounts in canola oil, soy oil, walnuts, ground flaxseed, soybeans and other nuts and seeds. Cold water fish, particularly salmon, mackerel, cod, herring, sardines, swordfish, and tuna are rich in omega-3 fatty acids. Eggs are another source of omega-3 fatty acids, though in lower amounts. Omega-3 fatty acids are referred to as either eicosapentaenoic acid (EPA) or docosahexaenoic acid (DHA). It has been suggested that 650 mg per day of an omega-3 fatty acid be consumed for proper maintenance of health; some have argued that intakes as high as 1,000 to 4,000 mg per day be achieved for optimal benefit.

While these potentially beneficial fatty acids are particularly high in swordfish and albacore tuna, these fish have been recently found to have relatively high and potentially dangerous concentrations of mercury and thus these types of fish should be completely avoided by women who are pregnant, nursing or who may become pregnant and young children. For others, these fish as well as shark, king mackerel, and tilefish should not be eaten more than twice a week with a total intake not to exceed 12 ounces. Some have suggested only using the "white" or "light" canned tuna if one is to use packaged varieties or the yellow-tail variety of tuna, available only in fresh form. Albacore tuna, commonly used in canned preparations, should be limited to one, six ounce portion or two, three ounce portions per week. The Environmental Protection Agency (EPA) reports low mercury levels in salmon, pollock, shrimp, canned light tuna, among many others and continues to recommend that seafood be incorporated into the diet for two meals a week.

Classification of Fatty Acids

Omega-3 fatty acids: fatty acids that are highly polyunsaturated and have a carbon-carbon double bond in the n-3 position. Studies have demonstrated that these have anti-inflammatory properties and may possibly reduce blood clotting in arteries and help prevent heart disease as well as improve cognition. These fatty acids are mostly derived from seafood and certain vegetable oils, nuts and seeds. Alpha- linolenic acid (ALA) is readily converted to an omega-3 fatty acid such as eicosapentaenoic acid (EPA) and docosahexaenoic acid (DHA).

Omega-6 fatty acids: fatty acids that are highly polyunsaturated and have a carbon-carbon double bond in the n-6 position. They are converted by the body to n-6 eicosanoids that bind to various receptors in the body and play a role in prostaglandin and leukotriene hormones. Linoleic acid and arachidonic acid are examples of omega-6 fatty acids. While these are also thought to help promote a healthy heart by lowering total and LDL cholesterol, they are considered to be pro-inflammatory and should not be consumed without at least three times as much omega-3 fatty acids being eaten at the same time. Vegetable oils, especially soybean, corn, and safflower are good sources of omega-6 fatty acids.

Trans fatty acids: This type of fatty acid is formed during the manufacturing process by hydrogenation of other fatty acids. Although they are found naturally in some foods, these are largely man-made and considered to act similar to saturated fats and raise LDL-cholesterol, the bad form of fat that circulates in the body, as well as reduce HDL-cholesterol, a fat that is cardiac protective. Hydrogenated fats are produced through the hydrogenation process. Studies have also demonstrated that trans fats are more likely to be converted to triglycerides by the liver and thus promote fat deposition and associated morbidity.

Fatty Acids: Characteristics and Benefits

Fatty acids are further characterized by their chemical structure and length. Saturated fatty acids that contain chain lengths from 8 to 10 carbons are referred to as medium-chain fatty acids. Longer-chain saturated fatty acids include lauric, myristic, palmitic, and stearic acids. Mono-unsaturated fatty acids include oleic acid and elaidic acid. The polyunsaturated fatty acids include linoleic acid and linolenic acid.

Individuals who consume diets low in total fat and rich in monounsaturated fatty acids and omega-3 fatty acids have the lowest rates of coronary artery disease. As stated previously, oils from cold water fish include the very-long-chain fatty acids, eicosapentaenoic acid, EPA, and docosahexaenoic acid, DHA, known as omega-3 oils. These fatty acids have several effects that are thought to be anti-atherogenic; they lower triglyceride levels, decrease platelet aggregation and clotting tendencies, and decrease inflammation. It is thought that these fatty acids incorporate into phospholipids and thus alter prostaglandin production and increase prostacyclin synthesis.

Studies have reported that men consuming 18 to 40 grams of omega-3 containing fish per day had a reduced mortality rate and a 25 to 65% reduction in coronary artery disease. One study in men who already had a myocardial infarction reported that an intake of 40 grams of omega-3 containing fish per day reduced mortality by 29%; these same authors, however, failed to demonstrate any reduction in the rate of men having a repeat heart attack.

The Inuit Eskimos are a prime example of the likely benefits of eating correctly. Despite the fact that these hardy natives eat a diet high in fat content and calories, they remain relatively healthy. Their diet is essential and provides a "metabolic" answer to help survive in cold climates; the "extra" body fat their diet promotes provides not only insulation from the cold but also helps maintain health despite the additional calorie requirements of dwelling in sub-zero weather. While one would argue that this high fat diet, in this case largely from coldwater fish and seal blubber, would promote heart disease, the data actually suggests the opposite in this select population. Further research on this has led to the conclusion that eating coldwater fish that are high in omega-3 fatty acids may be providing protection to the Eskimos and perhaps others who eat a diet of similar content. Clearly, this is only part of the story with significant physical activity, genetic make-up, and lifestyle also obviously playing a key role.

Just how do omega-3 fatty acids work to reduce heart disease if this is true? Several possible reasons include:

1. Reduced platelet aggregation and thus less of a chance to form a thrombus that blocks blood flow to areas of the heart.
2. Reduced levels of C-reactive protein, a marker for inflammation. High levels of C-reactive protein have been linked to the development of heart disease and rupture of plaques within the coronary vessels; this leads to vessel obstruction and myocardial infarction.

3. Reduced inflammation in blood vessels themselves due to anti-oxidant properties and thus less chance for endothelial damage within the vessels supplying blood to the heart.
4. Improved function of endothelial cells, the cells that line blood vessels and thus healthier and more resistant blood vessels.
5. Increased nitric oxide synthesis leading to vasodilation of the blood vessels supplying blood to the heart.
6. Reduced blood pressure and thus improved cardiac performance and less chance of damage to the vessels.
7. Reduced triglyceride and LDL-cholesterol levels.

There appears to be benefit even after heart disease has been established. Patients with chronic heart failure have been shown to benefit from taking n-3 polyunsaturated fatty acids (n-3 PUFA). Patients taking a one gram supplement of n-3 PUFA as compared to those given a placebo had a reduced risk for death and hospitalization for cardiovascular reasons regardless of their cause of heart failure, severity of illness, age, left ventricular ejection fraction, presence of diabetes, or cholesterol level.

One landmark study provides evidence of yet another possible benefit from consuming a diet high in omega-3 fatty acids. In the 1990's, a group of Dutch researchers reported that omega-3 fatty acid consumption was inversely related to the development of dementia, particularly Alzheimer's disease. In fact, high intake of total fat, saturated fat and cholesterol have all been demonstrated to increase the risk of developing dementia in later life with total fat intake having the highest correlation.

A Dutch group of investigators evaluated over 1,600 subjects aged 45 to 70 over a ten year period of time. These authors used a variety of neuropsychological testing parameters to measure cognition including memory and psychomotor response time in relation to fat consumption. Of the nine categories of dietary fats that were measured, diets that were high in saturated fatty acids and cholesterol were associated with an "increased" risk of cognitive decline. Consumption of diets high in fatty fish and omega-3 fatty acids (combined intake of DHA and EPA), however, were associated with a reduced risk of cognitive decline. Other fats including monounsaturated fatty acids, polyunsaturated fatty acids, alpha-linolenic acid (an omega-3 fatty acid precurser), linoleic acid (an omega-6 fatty acid), and total fat each taken separately had no significant effect on cognition. Clearly, additional research is warranted to better determine the role of these fatty acids in promoting health and helping to ward off disease.

Dementia is a syndrome with multiple causes including small strokes that may result from bleeding into key areas of the brain or thrombotic events caused by blood clots traveling through the brain's vessels and blocking blood flow to healthy brain tissue; accumulation of "plaques with a central amyloid protein core" and "neurofibrillary tangles" resulting in the illness known as

Alzheimer's disease; or a variety of treatable and even preventable causes including medication side-effects, depression, metabolic problems, sensory defects, nutritional problems such as vitamin B12 and folic acid deficiency, normal pressure hydrocephalus, tumors, trauma, infections, and alcoholism. Exactly what resulted in the benefit in cognition that was observed remains unknown but is clearly worthy of further investigation.

It is also worth noting that DHA levels have been positively correlated with levels of dopamine and serotonin, both implicated in our regulation of mood and a target of antidepressant drug therapy. In animals, a low level of DHA has been linked to symptoms of depression though no data is available to make this same conclusion in human subjects at this time. Omega-3 fatty acids may impact our mood as well as our physical well-being.

Not all fatty acids are created equal and some may actually be harmful. Saturated fatty acids raise serum triglyceride levels, total cholesterol, LDL-cholesterol, and have variable effects on HDL-cholesterol. This is a result of the effects of lauric, myristic and palmitic acids; stearic acid has little or no effect on serum lipids. Trans-fatty acids raise LDL-cholesterol levels and produce a small lowering of HDL and are considered to be harmful. Dietary cholesterol is capable of raising serum total cholesterol with 80 to 90% of the increase being in the form of LDL-cholesterol and a slight increase in HDL-cholesterol levels.

Effect of Dietary Fat on Blood Lipids

Type of fat/fatty acids	Effect on blood lipids
Saturated	Increased total cholesterol, increased LDL cholesterol
Polyunsaturated	Decreased total cholesterol, decreased LDL cholesterol, decreased HDL cholesterol
Monounsaturated	Decreased total cholesterol, decreased LDL cholesterol, increased or no effect on HDL cholesterol
Omega-3	Decreased triglycerides, decreased total cholesterol
Trans	Increased total cholesterol, increased LDL cholesterol, decreased or no effect on HDL cholesterol

While polyunsaturated fats are considered to be healthier than saturated fats, monounsaturated fats, such as olive oil and canola oil, are considered to be most heart healthy. Monounsaturated fatty acids are neutral on serum total cholesterol levels but have been shown to lower the level of LDL-cholesterol, long thought to be the "bad" form of cholesterol while raising the good form of cholesterol, HDL

While most of the positive attention regarding the benefits of monounsaturated fat comes from data relating to olive oil, studies have shown similar if not improved benefit from canola oil use. Canola oil is derived from the rape seed and originally was imported from Canada and thus the name "Can ola". Despite the relatively high fat content in diets of individuals living in the Mediterranean region, heart disease was noted to be less common as compared to that of persons consuming an American diet where saturated and polyunsaturated fats were more common. Studies demonstrated that not all fats were equivalent and thus the conclusion that we should be consuming more monounsaturated fats. Studies have not advocated for more fat in the diet, but rather have shown that if ingested in equal amounts, those who consumed olive or canola oil had a better lipid profile and perhaps a reduced rate of heart disease.

The consumer must beware, however, as they may easily fall prey to marketing that suggests certain fats are healthy merely because they are derived from "vegetable oils". Palm and coconut oil, for example, are both highly saturated and anything but heart healthy. For years, we were also led to believe that margarine was "safer" than butter. Butter, being an animal fat is saturated; margarine is usually derived from vegetable oils that are polyunsaturated. The hydrogenation process, however, changes the structure of fat making it more saturated. As a result of this alteration in composition, oils become semisolid and more stable at room temperature. The manufacturers like to use this form of fat as it also extends the shelf life of foods and prevents the development of bad odors and rancid flavor. Hydrogenating certain oils may also change the consistency of the product such as occurs with peanut oil in peanut butter; the oil that is hydrogenated now remains mixed in the peanut butter and does not separate as occurs with naturally produced peanut butter.

Usually hydrogenation is only partial with a final product being between 5 and 60% saturated. These substances are referred to as trans fatty acids. These partially hydrogenated oils, even if they originally were derived from 100% vegetable oils, loose their health benefit and may even be dangerous, with some data suggesting that they may even increase the risk of developing cancer, not to mention the increased risk of heart disease that they have clearly been linked to. Trans fatty acids act like saturated fats and are capable of elevating LDL cholesterol while reducing HDL cholesterol levels. The federal government now mandates that all food manufacturers clearly label the amount of trans fats that a food contains though the consumer often has a hard time deciphering what the labels actually mean. Certain States and cities in the United States have already banned restaurants from using trans fats, leaving it up to the local chef to determine how to create various recipes. Unfortunately, palm oil or lard, both relatively high in saturated fat, are cheap substitutes and are increasingly being used as an alternative to trans fats in the food or cooking process.

Percent Saturated, Polyunsaturated and Monounsaturated Fat

Oil	% Saturated	% Poly-unsaturated	% Mono-unsaturated
Canola	6	32	62
Saffflower	9	26	65
Safflower	9	78	13
Flaxseed	10	28	62
Sunflower	12	69	19
Corn	13	59	28
Peanut	14	32	50
Soybean	15	61	24
Olive	17	11	72
Cottonseed	26	55	20
Lard	42	10	48
Beef fat	46	4	47
Palm	50	10	40
Butterfat	63	3	34
Coconut	92	2	6

An excessive amount of fat in the diet is not only unhealthy for the heart, but has been implicated in a higher rate of breast, colon, prostate, and pancreatic cancers. Recent data has implicated dietary fat consumption during adolescence as an important modifiable risk factor for the development of breast cancer. While there remains controversy as to whether fat in the diet increases the risk of developing breast cancer, data derived from the Nurses' Health Study, 1 and 11, suggest that a greater consumption of vegetable fat during high school possibly protected girls against the development of breast cancer years later with up to a 39% reduction in risk as compared to those consuming a similar amount of animal fat.

This study involved over 120,000 nurses in its first cohort collected in 1976; a second cohort of 116,000 women was enrolled in 1989. Women enrolled in the Nurses' Health Study 11 aged 26 to 46 were also found to have an association between increased breast cancer risk and a greater intake of dietary animal fat. Some argue that this results from high levels of progesterone found in cow's milk, a source of fat derived from animals. Retrospective studies from Greece and Italy also point to a possible association between a greater consumption of olive oil and reduced risk of developing breast cancer.

Cholesterol is only one component of fat in the diet. While the maximum suggested daily intake should not exceed 300 mg of cholesterol, many suggest much lower levels in order to protect against heart disease. It is important to remember, however, that the body produces cholesterol and that even if one were to eliminate cholesterol in the diet completely, there may still be a high level found in one's blood. There is a definite correlation between serum cholesterol levels and levels of cholesterol in the diet. This relationship, however, is not always that simple as our bodies make cholesterol through a series of metabolic pathways in the liver even without any dietary intake. Under normal conditions, we have certain genes that help us regulate our enzymes in order to determine just how much cholesterol we have circulating in our bodies. If we take in more cholesterol than we need, our bodies "down regulate" cholesterol production and thus our levels drop to a desirable and safe level. Unfortunately, some of us lack the normal regulatory mechanisms and will continue to produce cholesterol even when our levels exceed what is considered to be safe. If we have an extreme case and lack all of the regulatory genes for monitoring and adjusting cholesterol in our bodies, we die early of heart disease. For the majority of us, however, we have varying abilities to maintain a balance with less dramatic, though still significant, effects on our cardiovascular system and health. Medications that have been developed to reduce LDL-cholesterol do so by altering cholesterol production in the liver through a variety of means.

It is important to remember that cholesterol is only part of the story of coronary artery disease with the lining of the blood vessels, the endothelium, first thought to have some form of damage as may result from hypertension, and then an accumulation of cellular debris, lipids, calcium, platelets, and fibrin each contributing and helping to create a narrowing and eventual closure of the vessel. This effectively results in an insufficient blood flow to tissues and an inability to maintain oxygen delivery to heart cells. This process slowly produces ischemia and eventually a myocardial infarction or heart attack. In certain circumstances, even small changes to the lining of the blood vessels of the heart fall prey to an acute accumulation of platelets and other cellular debris and cause the vessel to close.

CHAPTER

11

Reducing the Risk of Cardiovascular Disease Through Diet and Lifestyle

Various nutrients have been demonstrated to have significant effects on cardio-vascular disease risk reduction. Cardiovascular disease risk is reduced by approximately 30% for every 200 mg/1,000 kcal/day that one is able to reduce one's cholesterol intake. For every 10 gram increase in dietary soluble fiber, the risk for cardiac events is thought to be reduced by approximately 20–25%.

Moderate consumption of alcohol has also been reported to have a benefi-cial effect in preventing cardiovascular disease. This potential benefit has been linked to the chemical resveratrol, a chemical compound found in the skins of certain grapes. Produced naturally by grapes to fight off fungal diseases that commonly affect grapes when they are damp, its content varies widely depend-ing on the type of grape, where it is grown, and how the wine is processed. Since resveratrol is found primarily on grape skins, it is almost non-existent in most white wines that are fermented after the grape skins have been removed. Even some mass produced red wines have little of this possibly life-extending chemical as the skins are filtered in the production process to remove tannins that may contribute to a "bitter" taste found in some wines.

The highest concentrations of resveratrol are reportedly found in pinot noir grapes that grow in cooler, rainy places such as the Finger Lake region of upstate New York and Oregon's Willamette Valley. Pinot noir is also grown in the Burgundy region of France and has been found to have as much as 40 times the amount of resveratrol as grapes used to make merlot and cabernet sauvignon.

Resveratrol is quite unstable and once a bottle of wine has been opened, its potency dissipates within one day. Certain grape juices have also been found to have relatively high concentrations of resveratrol and may have a similar beneficial effect. Most commercially available grape juices unfortunately contain a wide variety of grapes, are frequently filtered in the manufacturing process, and supplemented with apple juice and undesirable sweeteners.

Resveratrol has been demonstrated to extend the life of yeast cultures and fruit flies and lower LDL cholesterol levels in humans while raising HDL cholesterol, the good form of cholesterol. Laboratory rats fed diets rich in resveratrol had significantly longer life-spans than those who were not and comparable to those fed low calorie diets that have been shown to extend their life-spans. In another series of experiments, salt-sensitive rats that had high blood pressure were fed a high-salt diet and a mixture of ground up grapes, equivalent to 9 servings of grapes a day. Improvements were noted in blood pressure. Another group of these rats were fed a diet low in salt and after 18 weeks of receiving a grape supplement were noted to not only have lower blood pressure than similar rats placed on the same diet but not given the mixture of powdered grapes, but were also noted to have improved heart muscle function and structure and lower levels of markers of inflammation. One study reported lower rates of lung cancer, particularly in persons who smoked, for individuals who consumed moderate quantities of red wine. Unfortunately, little human data are available upon which to draw any definitive conclusions at this time.

While one to two glasses of red wine, particularly pinot noir, or red grape juice per day may help reduce cardiovascular risk, it is important to remember that this finding remains controversial. Since higher intake of alcohol has been clearly linked to a myriad of health problems such as hepatitis, cirrhosis, pancreatitis, cardiomyopathy, increased esophageal and head and neck cancers among many other illnesses, caution is advised prior to increasing alcohol use. Alcohol also contains a relatively high amount of calories, 7 kcal per gram.

As stated previously, omega-3 fatty acids may offer protection from heart disease and may offer other health benefits as well. Individuals who consume 30 to 40 grams per day of cold water fish as compared to those who have little or no fish in their diet reportedly have 35% less cardiovascular disease.

If one is able to increase serum levels of folate from less than 6.8 micromols/liter to more than 13.6 micromols/liter, there is reportedly a 38% heart disease risk reduction; this is similar to that achieved by reducing one's serum homocysteine level by 5 micromols. This benefit is thought to be due to a prevention of thrombosis or aggregation of platelets and not through an effect on serum lipids.

Even Vitamin E has been linked to a reduced risk of cardiovascular disease with a 35% risk reduction noted for individuals taking 200–400 IU per day as compared to individuals with intakes of only 3–6 IU daily. This may be due to vitamin E's anti-oxidant effect, its role as an anti-inflammatory agent, and/or its role in helping to produce omega-3 fatty acids.

Clearly diet can be a very powerful adjunct to a regular exercise regimen. Physical activity 5 to 7 times per week has been shown to reduce cardiovascular risk by as much as 50% with benefits thought to be secondary to its ability to lower blood pressure and levels of low density lipoproteins, or the "bad" form of cholesterol, and increase HDL levels, the good form of cholesterol. In addition, exercise improves cardiac muscle performance similar to the effect one sees with other muscles that are stimulated as part of a physical fitness program. Muscle cells hypertrophy, or become larger, and recent data also suggests that heart cells may proliferate in response to various stimuli. Physical activity is also an excellent adjunct to a diet and promotes weight loss by increasing caloric expenditure. Since muscle is the major determinant of our metabolic activity, increased muscle mass resulting from exercise increases our metabolic rate and thus improves our caloric efficiency and metabolic balance.

As mentioned above, exercise promotes high levels of HDL-cholesterol, thought to be protective against heart disease. Despite data that shows a positive effect of higher HDL-cholesterol on preventing heart disease, physicians still look at the absolute level of LDL-cholesterol as the most important risk factor and strive to have it within a suitable range even if the HDL-cholesterol level is high. The average HDL level for men is between 40 and 50 mg/dl and for women 50 to 60. Recent data suggest that both men and women should strive to maintain their HDL levels above 60 gm/dl. HDL-cholesterol levels may be lowered by a variety of factors including insulin resistance, elevated triglycerides, obesity, physical inactivity, high carbohydrate intakes (>60% of calories), and certain medications including beta-blockers, anabolic steroids, and progestational agents.

The American Heart Association has recently lowered its threshold for starting cholesterol-lowering medications. It is important to remember that diet still plays a significant role in management even if these medications have been started.

LDL-cholesterol levels above 190 mg/dl are considered very high and in need of reduction even if there is no history of heart disease and no other risk factors. While some would still attempt diet and exercise, cholesterol-lowering drug therapies are currently being recommended earlier in these cases by the American Heart Association; some experts suggest making 160 mg/dl the threshold for starting pharmacologic treatment though not all agree as medications may have their own set of side-effects and in rare circumstances can be life-threatening.

Individuals with existing heart disease or diabetes are considered to be at highest risk and should aim for an LDL of less than 100 mg/dl; some have suggested that this value is still too high and have suggested a goal of 70 mg/ml. Levels greater than this should trigger a thorough review of one's diet and lifestyle and modification made immediately. LDL levels above 130 mg/dl deserve to be treated with lipid lowering medications in these high risk individuals while diet and lifestyle modification are allowed to take effect. In some, medication may be able to be eliminated over time. Some authorities believe that even levels between 100 and 129 mg/dl require early use of medication in those at highest risk.

Individuals with two or more risk factors for cardiac disease should maintain their LDL-cholesterol levels less than 130 mg/dl. Individuals with a LDL-cholesterol greater than 130 mg/dl should immediately initiate lifestyle changes and diet management as the 10 year risk of a cardiac event if left untreated is between 10 and 20%. If your LDL is greater than 130 after three months on a diet and exercise program, drug treatment may need to be started.

Individuals with no or one risk factor should maintain an LDL-cholesterol level below 160 mg/dl. Higher levels mandate diet and lifestyle modification and levels greater than 190 mg/dl will likely require medication. Between 160 and 189 mg/dl there is room for individualized consideration with heavy use of cigarettes, very low levels of HDL-cholesterol, and strong family history useful in helping to determine if someone should be started on medicines earlier.

Once again, there is considerable debate even in the medical profession as to exactly when someone should be started on a statin medication to lower cholesterol levels. Since these medications are not without complete risk, there is still room for interpretation and individual choice.

Major risk factors that must be considered when determining whether a specific level of LDL-cholesterol may be appropriate include:

- Use of cigarettes

- Hypertension (BP > or equal to 140/90 mmHg or anyone already on anti-hypertensive medication)

- Low HDL cholesterol (<40 mg/dl)

- Family history of premature heart disease, e.g. male first-degree relative under 55 years and/or female first degree relative under age 65

- Age (men >45 and women >55)

- Diabetes, other forms of atherosclerotic disease such as peripheral arterial disease, abdominal aortic aneurysm and symptomatic carotid artery disease are considered an equivalent risk to existing cardiovascular disease

Cholesterol-lowering medications are not without complete risk with damage to the liver and muscles reported as the most significant potential side-effects. Lifestyle modification is key regardless of one's LDL-cholesterol level. Weight management, exercise, stress reduction, and proper diet help everyone. If one is trying to use diet to treat an elevated LDL-cholesterol level, cholesterol intake should be reduced below 200 mg/day and saturated fat should be limited to no more than 7% of total calorie intake at least until one reaches their established goal. After this a more liberal use of saturated fat may be allowed but never should it exceed 10% of total calories with total fat limited to no more than 30%. Fiber, especially soluble fiber should be increased with the goal being an intake of over 25 grams per day.

Diets have a beneficial effect in helping to prevent heart disease by not only reducing cholesterol and fat intake in the diet but also by causing a negative calorie balance and thus a reduction in weight. As we loose weight, we loose both muscle and fat content in the body. Thus the need to exercise whenever we are on a diet as this will help maintain our muscle mass and shift the weight loss in favor of loosing more fat. In fact, as we loose weight, we also change the size of our fat cells. As fat cells become smaller, they become more sensitive to the action of insulin and in time, our insulin levels decline helping to further reduce our risk of developing heart problems.

Studies have shown that maintaining higher levels of insulin throughout the day, not just in response to meals (a normal process that serves to drive blood sugar into cells to produce energy), increases our risk for the development of heart disease.

Data from animal studies demonstrate that when insulin is allowed to rise in response to meals and drop to a basal level when not needed to drive sugar into cells, there is a "permissive" or positive effect in preventing atherogenesis; estrogen given to these animals had a protective effect against the development of heart disease. When insulin was manipulated to remain higher than normal throughout the day and not allowed to fall as it would normally do after a meal, estrogen no longer had a protective effect and the animal had more heart and vascular disease.

The Paris Prospective Study evaluated over 7,000 Paris policemen over a 15 year time span measuring many factors including results of a glucose tolerance test that measured insulin response to blood sugar. They concluded that the response that individuals had to a blood sugar challenge in terms of insulin elevation correlated years later to the development of heart disease. In other words, those individuals who had the highest insulin response to a blood sugar challenge, had the most heart disease many years later.

Clearly this has implications for treatment. Individuals who are overweight or obese maintain higher levels of basal insulin than those who are thin. This higher insulin level may have significant unwanted consequences; if fat cells were smaller and more sensitive to the action of insulin, as occurs with weight loss, the insulin levels would drop to a more normal and safe level. The use of complex-carbohydrates have also been shown to increase the sensitivity of tissues to the action of insulin, effectively causing insulin levels to be lower and more conducive to proper health.

Insulin insensitivity or insulin resistance leads to a state that has been named Metabolic Syndrome or Syndrome X. This Syndrome has been associated with a greater risk of developing heart disease and diabetes and requires immediate treatment. The following are criteria for defining who has Metabolic Syndrome; individuals who have any three of the following meet the definition in a pure sense though most persons with this are obese, have abnormally high lipid levels, and high blood pressure.

1. Men who have a waist circumference greater than 102 cm or 40 inches and women who have a waist circumference greater than 88 cm or 35 inches
2. Triglyceride levels greater than 150 mg/dl
3. HDL-cholesterol levels less than 40 mg/dl for men and 50 mg/dl for women
4. Blood pressure greater than 130/85 mmHg
5. Fasting blood glucose greater than 110 mg/dl

Underlying causes should be promptly treated such as physical inactivity and/or obesity. Blood pressure should be treated and LDL-cholesterol levels reduced to the desired goal by whatever means necessary. Aspirin use is suggested for those with existing coronary artery disease to reduce the prothrombotic state that commonly occurs and dietary adjustments should be made to reduce elevated triglycerides and/or low HDL levels if present. Elevated triglyceride levels usually respond to dietary adjustment and weight loss. If the triglycerides remain high, medication may be required with the goal of achieving levels of less than 150 mg/dl.

Any person with an elevated LDL-cholesterol or other form of lipid abnormality should be evaluated to make sure that there is no other underlying cause or a "secondary dyslipidemia". This may be seen in individuals with any of the following disorders: Diabetes mellitus, hypothyroidism, obstructive liver disease, chronic renal failure, and use of medications that may increase LDL-cholesterol and reduce HDL-cholesterol levels such as anabolic steroids, corticosteroids, and progestins.

Lastly, stress, either real or perceived, is a risk factor for the development of many illnesses including hypertension, cardiovascular and cerebrovascular disease, ulcers, among others. There are many techniques that can be followed to reduce "stress" in our everyday lives, many of which can be self-taught and mastered (See Chapter 17: The Mind-Body Connection and Its Role in Reducing Stress).

12

The Role of Protein in Successful Aging

The body requires a continuous intake of protein to replace amino acids that have been lost. Protein is also capable of supplying your body with energy if you fail to eat sufficient carbohydrates and fats. Proteins are a component of every cell, organ, and tissue in the body. They are made up of building blocks, or amino acids, each with a unique structure and function and consist of carbon, hydrogen, and oxygen. Your body uses 20 amino acids to make proteins. In fact, it is the amino acid patterns in the proteins that determine the characteristics of our tissues.

During times of growth, such as infancy, childhood, adolescence, and pregnancy, the body needs proteins to make new body tissues. Otherwise, proteins are used to build and repair body tissue. When you consume more protein than you need, it is broken down and stored as fat in the body and no longer serves as a reservoir for protein. Since there is no storage form of protein, proteins and other nitrogen containing compounds are degraded and resynthesized continuously. Proteins also help regulate the physiological way our bodies function through enzymes and hormones distributed throughout the body; these serve as vital catalysts for the various chemical reactions that are essential for proper health and well-being.

Protein in our diet serves as the source of the 20 amino acids found throughout the body. Nine of these amino acids (tryptophan, histidine, lysine, leucine, isoleucine, valine, threonine, phenylalanine, and methionine) are essential for humans and cannot be synthesized by the body. Histidine is particulary essential during periods of growth and development and can be produced in limited quantities. There is controversy as to whether histidine is an "essential" amino acid that must be in the diet after childhood. Cystine is synthesized from methionine; tyrosine is produced from its precursor, phenylalanine. The other amino acids are able to be produced by the body and are referred to as "non-essential" amino acids.

Most of the amino acids are metabolized within the liver. Valine, leucine and isoleucine, known as "branched amino acids", are degraded largely within peripheral tissues, such as skeletal muscle. They are also metabolized to a lesser degree within the kidney and fat where this process is coupled to the release of glutamine and alanine. These amino acids serve as carriers of ammonia and travel to the liver where nitrogen, a component of ammonia, can be converted into urea. During periods of significant caloric deprivation, these amino acids play a role in glucose production through a process known as gluconeogenesis. Glycine, valine, cystine, serine, aspartic acid, asparagines, threonine, methionine, glutamine, glutamic acid, praline, arginine, and histidine may also play a role in energy production by the body. Leucine and lysine are ketogenic amino acids and can produce acetyl coenzyme A (C0A) or acetoacetate, both involved in other energy producing metabolic pathways. Tyrosine, phenylalanine, and isoleucine are partially ketogenic with only a component of their carbon atoms being used in this process.

Aromatic amino acids serve as precursors for hormone production. Tryptophan is converted into serotonin while tyrosine serves as a basic component of thyroid hormone (thyroxine or T4) and the catecholamines (norepinephrine and epinephrine).

The recommended dietary allowance for protein has been established at 0.8 grams per kg body weight. While most individuals can tolerate up to twice this amount for short amounts of time without any undesirable consequences, a long-term effect of eating too much protein may be an accelerated decline in our kidney function. While data in humans is not available, experiments in animals have demonstrated that high protein intake increases pressure within the kidney leading to an increase in inflammation and scarring and a reduction in kidney function over time. There is no reason to expect that the human kidney would act differently and thus some have advocated for lowering the protein recommendation in our diet to 0.6 grams/kilogram of body weight. High amounts of protein in the diet, particularly if derived from animal sources, additionally can lead to increased demineralization of our bones. Individuals with abnormal kidney or liver function must clearly have more restricted protein content in their diet to avoid side effects resulting from high levels of ammonia produced when protein is degraded.

Proteins can be obtained from numerous food sources. Meat, poultry, fish, eggs, milk, cheese, yogurt, and soy provide all nine essential amino acids and are referred to as "complete" proteins. Legumes (beans and peas), seeds, and nuts are considered to be "nearly" complete proteins as they contain almost all of the nine essential amino acids. Grain products and many vegetables provide protein, though if taken alone lack one or more essential amino acids and are referred to as "incomplete" proteins.

Vegetarians are often considered to be at risk of consuming either insufficient or inadequate quantities of protein. Except for fruit, almost every food of plant origin contains at least some protein with nuts, seeds and legumes having the highest amount. Incomplete sources of protein are easily complemented when mixed with other incomplete proteins. To obtain complete protein, however, there is no need to combine specific foods at each meal as was once thought to be necessary. Our bodies are amazingly adept at utilizing what is consumed throughout the day to make its "own" complete proteins. Whatever amino acid one food or meal lacks can easily be derived from some other food consumed throughout the day. Vegetarians who consume dairy and egg products should have no problem obtaining all essential nutrients including the necessary essential amino acids. If protein quality is questioned in the diet, vegetarians may need to consume a higher protein content than the minimum requirement; nevertheless, a varied plant-based diet if appropriately planned provides sufficient protein in most circumstances. Those persons who are in doubt should consult a dietitian for advice.

Vegan diets contain no foods of animal origin including dairy products. For this reason, vegans need to be more cautious and may need to also consider using a vitamin and mineral supplement. They are more frequently at risk of developing deficiencies in Vitamin B12, Vitamin D, calcium, iron and zinc.

Gluten is a composite of the proteins gliadin and glutenin and comprises 80% of the protein contained in wheat seed. While a good source of protein, it is lacking certain essential amino acids and thus must be used with other protein sources to meet one's complete amino acid needs. Being insoluble in water, gluten proteins can be purified easily by washing away the associated starch and throughout the world gluten is an important source of protein. Food can be prepared directly from sources containing gluten or it can be added to foods otherwise low in protein. While corn and rice also contain proteins that are sometimes referred to as glutens, their proteins lack glutenin, the component in wheat flour that gives kneaded dough its elasticity, allows leavening and gives the chewiness to baked products. Seitan is a vegan meat substitute that is derived from cooking wheat gluten. High in protein and low in carbohydrate, seitan is usually made by combining "vital wheat gluten" with water and either boiling or baking the mixture. Both gluten and seitan are used in a variety of dishes, usually stir frys, and are frequently mixed with vegetables and spices as they both take on a variety of flavors depending on how they are used.

While any protein source that provides all of the essential amino acids can promote health and the ability of the body to build muscle mass, the bodybuilding literature is replete with data suggesting that Whey Protein more readily helps heal muscle injury and promote muscle formation. Whey protein is a collection of proteins isolated from whey, a by-product of cheese manufactured from cow's milk. It is a mixture of various globular proteins consisting typically of 65% beta-lactoglobulin, 25% alpha-lactalbumin, and 8% serum albumin. Whey has the highest biological value of any known protein and is considered to be extremely digestible. Whey protein is commonly used by athletes and bodybuilders to accelerate the formation of muscle mass and promote necessary healing. Some individuals use whey protein to increase their antioxidant levels as it is an excellent dietary source of cysteine, an essential amino acid and the rate-limiting factor in the production of glutathione, a potent antioxidant. While it is an excellent source of protein, whey supplements may also help prevent the rapid up and down shifts of blood sugar following the ingestion of carbohydrates.

13

The Role of Carbohydrates in Health and Disease

We often hear the terms "low carb", "high carb", "good carbs" and "bad carbs". What do these terms actually refer to? Carbohydrates consist of sugars and complex carbohydrates. The sugars include the monosaccharides such as glucose and fructose, and disaccharides such as sucrose, maltose, and lactose or milk sugar. Complex carbohydrates are polysaccharides and comprise starches and fiber. Starches consist of glucose built together as a polymer. Fibers are mainly indigestible complex carbohydrates that come from plant cell walls, such as cellulose, hemicellulose, and pectin and a variety of mucilages, gums, and algal polysaccharides. Lignin is a non-carbohydrate component of dietary fiber found in plant cell walls. Once eaten, dietary fibers are converted into absorbable fatty acids by intestinal microorganisms. Pentoses and organic acids such as citric and malic acids and a number of polyols including xylitol and sorbitol are also considered to be carbohydrates.

The average American eats half of their carbohydrates in the form of monosaccharides and disaccharides as are found in fruits and milk. Sugars are most commonly found in soft drinks, candy, jams, jellies, and desserts and mainly consist of sucrose and high-fructose corn syrup. While perhaps good for the farm economy, corn syrup has become an all too often used sweetener. Studies have found an association between consumption of high-fructose corn syrup containing foods and a number of medical conditions including fatty liver disease, kidney disease with protein in the urine, obesity, and diabetes. Some argue that fructose is more quickly converted to fat than other sugars by bypassing the body's normal metabolic pathways.

Complex carbohydrates consist largely of starches such as cereal grains, potatoes, legumes, and other vegetables. Sugars and starches provide a major portion of energy in the diet. Glucose is absorbed in the intestine or produced by the liver through a process known as gluconeogenesis and is a major component of energy production by the body. Fructose and galactose are converted into glucose in the liver. Glucose can also be derived from amino acids, glycerol components of fat and some organic acids and thus carbohydrates are not "essential" for energy production. Without carbohydrates in the diet, however, energy from lipolysis or the breakdown of stored triglycerides and the oxidation of fatty acids increase and ketone bodies accumulate. Protein can also be broken down and used to produce energy.

While there is no "amount" of carbohydrates in the diet that actually defines whether one's diet is "low" or "high" in carbohydrate content, most individuals consuming a "normal" American diet consume between 40 and 60% of their calories in the form of carbohydrate. Those who want to increase their intake of carbohydrates in the diet usually push carbohydrates to over 65% of total calories. The bad carbs are the "refined" starches and sugars such as that found in white bread, white pasta and other white flour products, sugar, candy, and most snack foods. These carbohydrates are easily broken down into sugar and result in rapid swings of both blood sugar and insulin levels. They tend to make one more hungry and over time result in excess calories being consumed; these are converted into fat and stored for future use. They also tend to more commonly result in fatigue, irritability, and even mood swings. Some have suggested that they may also be associated with attention deficit disorders in both children and adults.

Good carbohydrates are considered to be "complex" and are found largely in whole grains, fruits, and vegetables. They contain more fiber and have benefit beyond their calories by helping to keep blood sugar more "even" throughout the day. These foods have also been shown to sensitize the tissues in the body to the action of insulin thus reducing levels of insulin and helping to promote a healthier metabolism.

Most people find it easier to eat an excessive amount of carbohydrates than other nutrients, a frequent reason given as to why we should proactively take steps to limit our carbohydrate intake. Perhaps this is due to the increased appetite we get from the higher levels of insulin that result from carbohydrate intake though there may be other reasons for this as well including psychological factors. Knowing this, it is essential to set an appropriate portion size ahead of the meal to prevent this from happening and allow the beneficial aspects of one's diet without eating to excess. People who eat diets that limit carbohydrates tend to consume less calories as it is harder to eat an excessive amount of fat and protein; since these latter foods stimulate insulin less effectively, there is less appetite stimulation. In fact, diets high in fat and protein if taken to an extreme tend to cause one to be anorectic due to the acidic environment that is created in our bodies referred to as "acidosis" as these are degraded.

While this may sound like a perfect solution, excess protein has been shown to cause an accelerated aging process for the kidneys in animals and a greater loss of bone mass. Individuals who switch to a high fat, high protein diet also tend to loose the benefit of this in terms of their weight management program after 6 months and after two years, are in fact worse off by some accounts than those who chose a more balanced diet in the first place. Once carbohydrates are added back to the diet, even if in less quantity than previously ingested, the "acidosis" is no longer present and all that is left is the high fat and protein with its unwanted effects. Lipid profiles are also harmed with an increase in LDL cholesterol. While a few months of almost any diet may be viewed as "worth it" if it results in the desired effect on one's weight, the long-term benefit must clearly outweigh any negative effects. You should always be as informed as possible as to what you are facing in terms of benefits and risks. What is most important, however, whether your goal is to loose weight or just find the "right diet", is finding the specific diet routine that works for you, promotes health, and can be incorporated into your life long term.

14

Tips to Achieve a Healthier Diet: Eat Smart

1. Divide one's desired daily calorie intake into 3, 4 or 5 meals. This helps prevent the body from thinking it is "starving" during long periods without food intake. This helps prevent a reduction in body metabolism as the body tries to conserve energy during periods of caloric deprivation and will maximize your metabolic state.

2. If you plan to reduce your calorie intake, make sure that you drink lots of water or non-caloric drinks while limiting the amount of caffeine. Since up to 50% of the fluid one ingests every day comes from "hydrated foods", reducing daily calorie intake may lead to dehydration. Fluid also helps maintain a feeling a fullness and for some, satisfies the "oral" need otherwise derived from eating. Caffeine may make you feel "awake" or "stimulated", but it may also increase your nervousness and cause you to eat more.

3. Low calorie snacks help keep appetite in check and can be a way to supplement one's nutrition. They also help satisfy the "oral urge" that some people have. Slices of celery, tomato, lettuce, and cucumber are all outstanding ways to fight that urge to eat foods with higher calorie and other possible harmful contents. Eliminate temptations in the home as well and substitute healthy alternatives.

4. While usually more expensive, organic foods are more likely to be free of pesticides, hormones, and antibiotics. Organic meat comes from animals that are specially raised and fed. These animals are fed grain and not given food containing components of other animals. Many are grown on outdoor pastures and fed only certified organic feed. Even here, make sure that you read labels carefully and do not assume everything listed as being organic is desirable.

5. Read ingredient labels on the foods you buy. Ingredients are listed in descending order in proportion to the amount that is contained within the package itself.

   Make sure you understand what is listed on food labels and beware of "number of servings" and content "per 100 grams" or "% of RDA". Know what you are eating!

6. Take careful note of the "suggested portion size". Just because a food is pre-packaged and appears to be a single serving, does not mean that the package contains only "one" portion. Multiply each of the ingredient listings (and calories) by the number of portions listed on the package to find out the total amount of each and then divide by how many servings you intend to consume.

7. Avoid foods that are high in saturated fat. Just because something is made with 100% vegetable oil does not mean it is healthy.

8. Low fat foods may be high in sugar and do not necessarily equate to low calorie. Read labels carefully!

9. Hydrogenated fats refer to the manufacturing process that "saturates" chemical bonds by adding hydrogen. This results in the production of trans fats that are unhealthy and are best avoided. Trans fats, even if derived from otherwise heart healthy oils, are no longer similar in content or benefit.

10. Avoid foods prepared with non-organic cottonseed oil due to its potentially high levels of pesticides.

11. Food additives may include nitrites, caffeine, saccharin and artificial coloring among others. Make sure you know what you are eating and what you need to avoid.

12. Sugar derived from sugar cane is not the only way food is sweetened. Fructose, fruit juice, corn syrup, honey, barley malt, maltose and dextrose are also commonly added as sugar substitutes and all have calories and raise blood sugar and insulin levels. Not all nutrients that sound "healthy" actually are!

13. Not all fish are of equal health benefit. Cold water fish, such as salmon, cod, sardines, and herring have the highest content of heart healthy omega-3 oils and are good to incorporate into the diet for 2 or 3 meals each week. Mercury has been found in certain fish such as shark, tile fish, king mackerel, swordfish, and even certain types of tuna and these fish should be consumed in limited quantities or avoided all together if one is pregnant, nursing, a child, or just concerned over one's health.

14. Certain foods have been linked to a more heart healthy diet. These include garlic, onions, oat bran, cold water fish, red wine in limited amounts and/or grape juice, almonds and walnuts, cranberries, and certain teas. While data supporting their benefit may not be scientifically proven without any doubt, there is little risk involved and perhaps a lot to gain from their use.

15. Certain foods contain high concentrations of anti-oxidants and are thought to promote health. These foods include raspberries, blueberries, and black-berries; spinach and kale; dark-skinned fruits such as red apples and nectarines; certain teas such as black, green and orange pekoe; among others. Anti-oxidants have been shown to have beneficial effects in preventing oxidative damage from "free-radicals" and may have beneficial anti-inflammatory effects as well.

16. Certain foods are claimed to lower cancer rates including cabbage, tomatoes, broccoli, soybeans, garlic, and green tea. While data is inconclusive, there is little harm in choosing to include these excellent foods in one's diet and there is always the potential for benefit if the studies prove to be correct.

17. Certain foods have been linked to healthier eyes including spinach, kale, collards, broccoli, swiss chard, peaches, carrots, persimmons, corn and fresh water fish. These are all good choices to include in one's diet though once again, more data is needed prior to making any definitive conclusions as to their benefit.

CHAPTER

15

Selected Foods:
Unexpected Benefits

Chocolate

- 0.5 ounce or 1 tbs baking chocolate contains 80 calories; 1.0 gram protein; 4.0 grams carbohydrate; 8 grams fat; 2.0 grams fiber.
- 0.5 ounce of semisweet chocolate contains 70 calories; 1.0 gram protein; 8.0 grams carbohydrate; 4.5 grams fat; 1.0 gram fiber.
- 0.5 ounce of dark chocolate contains 70 calories; 1.0 gram of protein; 8.0 grams of carbohydrate; 4.0 grams of fat; 1.0 gram fiber.

Chocolate is made from cocoa beans found within the pods of the cacao tree. While many crave this food and enjoy its decadent texture and flavor, most fear its fat and relatively high calorie content. Interestingly, chocolate may not be all that bad and in fact has several redeeming and even health promoting qualities that may prove beneficial if taken in small amounts.

The Olmec people, an ancient tribe which lived centuries ago in Central America, were the first known individuals to make a water based drink from cocoa beans. Mixed with dried chilis and other native ingredients, this drink was referred to as kakawa and was thought to enhance one's "love making". In fact, Montezuma, the famous Aztec king, was said to drink this potion before retiring to his harem.

The cacao tree itself was named *Theobroma cacao*, or "food of the gods" by the famous Swedish botanist Linnaeus. Storytellers claim that Casanova was known to consume chocolate before entertaining his many paramours. According to a study published in the American Journal of Clinical Nutrition in 2000, chocolate has been found to contain high amounts of the antioxidant polyphenol, similar to that found in red wine and tea. Polyphenols are thought to protect one from heart disease by reducing the oxidation of low-density lipoproteins or bad cholesterol. Polyphenols also inhibit blood platelet aggregation, thought responsible for the occlusion of coronary arteries increasing one's risk of having a myocardial infarction. Studies have also reported that cocoa is capable of "thinning the blood" or reducing the time it takes to coagulate blood. Subjects given a concentrated cocoa beverage had lower platelet aggregation and took a longer time to form a clot. Cocoa in other words had the same beneficial effect as aspirin, long thought to be protective against heart attacks.

Individuals who consume dark chocolate also have higher levels of epicatechin, a beneficial antioxidant. Dark chocolate has been shown to improve lipid profiles in addition to its beneficial effects on platelet aggregation. Researchers have also demonstrated a beneficial effect from eating dark chocolate on blood pressure. When individuals with "mild hypertension" ate 100 grams of dark chocolate for two weeks in place of other foods with similar nutrients and calories, a significant drop in blood pressure, averaging 5 mm Hg systolic and 2 mm Hg diastolic, was noted. Those who ate white chocolate failed to have this effect.

I was pleased to have the opportunity to collaborate on a study with Drs. Paul Gurbel, Miruais Hamed, and others to study the effect of dark chocolate on platelet activity, C-Reactive Protein — a measure of our inflammatory processes — and the "good" and "bad" forms of cholesterol. Our data demonstrated that seven days of ingesting 100 grams of dark chocolate that provided 700 mg of flavonoids per day lowered LDL-cholesterol, the harmful form of cholesterol, by an average of 6% and raised HDL-cholesterol, the good form of cholesterol, by an average of 9%, both statistically significant changes. Measures of platelet aggregation were significantly reduced as well, implying less potential for thrombosis and cardiovascular risk. Of note, dark chocolate also significantly reduced C-Reactive Protein levels in the women in our study, implying a reduced state of inflammation; we did not find similar results in our men subjects. While this study had only 28 subjects, the findings were significant and clear in their message. Unfortunately, the calories provided in the dark chocolate are not insignificant and any weight gain and change in metabolism that might result from this ingestion if continued over time, would have their own negative effects. Finding out ways to achieve the positive effects of the dark chocolate whether due to the flavonoids alone or some other factor in the chocolate itself without potentially causing harm due to the indirect result of the added calories is well worth pursuing.

Since 100 grams of dark chocolate contains approximately 480 calories, it is not something that can in itself justify the high calories, especially since there are other ways to obtain equivalent beneficial nutrients without the added calories. For those who "crave" a chocolate fix, however, a "small portion" of dark chocolate may just be enough to provide a satisfying snack without the guilt.

Chocolate also contains hundreds of chemical compounds including phenylethylamine or PEA. This chemical has been found to stimulate the body's release of endorphins, a hormone that is part of our endogenous or natural "opioid system" and a possible mediator of the orgasmic response. Chocolate may potentiate the activity of dopamine, a neurochemical that serves an important role in the nervous system and is necessary for normal body movement and coordination. Dopamine is also thought to play a role in memory function and has been associated with sexual arousal. Of note, phenylethylamine has been found in higher amounts during orgasm and interestingly, higher amounts have reportedly also been found in individuals during the process of "falling in love".

Chocolate increases serotonin levels, possibly helping to explain at least in part the emotionally satisfying feeling many describe after eating chocolate. Anandamide is another chemical that is found in chocolate; its name is derived from the Sanskrit word ananda, which means "bliss". This chemical binds to the same receptor in the brain as the psychotropic ingredients of marijuana, the cannabinoids.

Clearly, there are many reasons why chocolate has earned its reputation as one of our favorite foods. Unfortunately, chocolate has a "bitter" flavor when unsweetened and few artificially sweetened varieties containing fewer calories yet with good taste have reached the market. Milk chocolate has the disadvantage of having an even higher calorie content than dark chocolate and milk appears to inactivate many of the antioxidants contained in the chocolate itself. For these reasons, dark chocolate is preferred though best reserved for that "special" occasion; even then, due to its high calorie content, it should only be eaten in small quantities. Good things can come in small sizes!

Cranberries

- 1/2 cup fresh berries contain 23 calories; 0 grams protein; 6.0 grams carbohydrate; 0 grams fat; 6.0 grams fiber.
- 8.0 ounces cranberry juice contains 60 calories; <1.0 gram protein; 14.0 grams carbohydrate; 0.0 grams fiber.

The name cranberry often brings memories of morning muffins or Thanksgiving relish. Cranberries are indeed much more and you may very well want to make them a part of your daily diet. Originally known to grow wild in bogs, cranberries were first formally characterized by the Swedish botanist Peter Kalm in 1749 who compared these to lingonberries, common to Sweden, but much larger in size. The scientific name for the cranberry species, Vaccinium macrocarpon, means "large fruit". The red fruit is also quite large in relation to the plant's small green leaves. Native to America, the cranberry was referred to by the Huron Indian tribe as "toca" or "atoca" meaning "good berry". The Wampanoag Indian tribe called them "ibimi, or "bitter berry" and the Narragansett Indians used the term "sasemineash" or "very sour berry".

Cranberries originally grew wild from Labrador to North Carolina and as far west as Minnesota. With the increase in population across America, however, fewer hospitable areas remain for their growth and they became more difficult to find even in these regions. Most commercially available cranberries now come from farms located in Massachusetts and Wisconsin. Cranberries prefer moist, acidic soil that is rich in organic matter.

Cranberry juice has been used by women with urinary tract infections for many years in the hope that its ability to acidify the urine will create a more hostile environment to infection causing bacteria. The truth is that one must consume a great deal of cranberry juice in order to achieve this potential benefit. Recently another potential benefit from drinking cranberry juice has been uncovered; drinking three, 8.0 ounce glasses of cranberry juice daily for a month was found to increase HDL cholesterol levels, the "good" form of cholesterol, by 10%. This is a significant factor in helping to protect against coronary artery disease. Studies have shown that for every milligram per deciliter that a person's HDL cholesterol rises, the risk of having a heart attack is reduced by approximately 3% for women and 2% for men. When coupled with other HDL elevating foods, such as oat bran, almonds, dark chocolate, and soy protein, and an exercise program that will also raise HDL levels, a measurable risk reduction is clearly within reach.

When taken in their natural form, cranberries are also an excellent source of fiber and antioxidants including Vitamin C. While natural cranberry juice is the logical choice, many find it too tart and prefer adding an artificial sweetener. Be careful of juice cocktails, however, that often contain high-fructose corn syrup and other sweeteners that provide empty calories and unnecessary carbohydrates.

Soy Protein

Soybeans have been cultivated and eaten in China for more than 2,000 years and Japanese diets have included soy products for centuries. Soy has been credited as being at least partially responsible for the Japanese being considered one of the healthiest and longest living populations on Earth. Besides being an excellent source of protein, soybeans also contain fiber, iron, calcium, folic acid, magnesium, potassium and B vitamins.

Soy is an excellent source of protein without the saturated fat and cholesterol found in protein derived from animals. Soy protein has been widely used throughout Asia in products such as soy milk, tofu, and tempeh and is quickly gaining acceptance in the US. Soy is increasingly being added to the US diet in the form of tofu and cereals are now adding soy protein to maximize their health benefit. Soy protein powder and energy bars are widely available and can provide a quick snack or even serve as a substitute for an entire meal. Soy nuts are also an excellent snack or supplement to a meal and edamame, the Japanese name for green soybeans, can be used as a healthy snack either steamed or uncooked or as a protein source as part of a healthy meal.

The first soybean crop in the US was planted in the Savannah, Georgia area in the 1700's. In fact, an enterprising Englishman even patented the formula for a "soy sauce". Soybeans were used during the Civil War as a substitute for coffee and in 1904, George Washington Carver, the African-American agricultural scientist, identified soybeans as an excellent source of protein and recommended that it be used as an oil. In the early 20th century, soybeans were commercially made into oil and advertised as an inexpensive source of protein. In fact, Dr. John Harvey Kellogg, the brother of the famous cereal manufacturer, was a vegetarian and developed soy as a meat substitute as early as the 1920's. During the difficult times of World War 2, soy again resurged as a protein source and various soy products were produced including burgers, cereals, and food substitutes. Despite this, soy failed to achieve wide acceptance until more recent times when a more positive Asian influence began to spread in the Western world. The first soy products to become widely accepted in the US were the soy based beverages, such as soymilk.

In 1995, a research study was published in the prestigious New England Journal of Medicine that revolutionized thinking about soy and its role in the western diet. This study for the first time determined that soy in the diet helped reduce blood cholesterol. By 1999, the US Food and Drug Administration agreed to allow food labels to state that there was a potential cholesterol-lowering effect from soy. The rest is history with soy quickly gaining popularity as an excellent source of protein and as a major source of phytoestrogens.

Soy protein is a "complete" protein and in fact is the only plant protein that is equivalent to animal protein in terms of its amino acid content. The US Department of Agriculture evaluates protein quality using the Protein Digestibility Corrected Amino Acids Score or PDCAAS. This effectively measures the amino acid pattern of proteins and factors in digestibility. Soy protein has a PDCAAS score of 1.0, equivalent to animal protein.

Everywhere we look, soy burgers are now ubiquitous and soy is even being added to breakfast cereals to enhance its health benefit.

Sales of soy have steadily increased in the US with close to a 14% increase annually from the early 1990's. Asians still consume more soy than the average American with intakes between 8 and 20 grams of soy protein per day not unusual; many feel that it is only a matter of time until the US diet catches up. There are currently over 3,000 food products containing soy available for the consumer, not to mention the availability of soy protein powder that can easily be added to any food either by sprinkling on top or through blending. Soy is now being added commercially to bread and other baked goods and soy-based meat alternatives are increasingly gaining popularity by mainstream America and in fact are made to be look-alikes of meat and poultry with texture and taste not much far behind. The average soy burger, for example, contains approximately 10 grams of soy protein, is generally free of cholesterol and saturated fat, and has a moderate sodium content. Soy is now available as a frozen dessert, an ice cream substitute, and as yogurt for the concerned health consumer.

Soy yogurt has a creamy texture and is easy to use as a substitute in recipes for sour cream or cream cheese. A soy cheese is also available that is made from soymilk. It also has a creamy texture that makes it a great substitute for most cheeses, sour cream, or cream cheese and it is also used as a topping on soy pizza. There is even a soy-based vodka manufactured by the 3 Vodka Distilling Company based in Chicago.

Soy has been shown to reduce total cholesterol, low-density lipoprotein (LDL) cholesterol, the "bad" cholesterol, and triglyceride levels, also potentially harmful to one's heart. This benefit occurs without a decrease in the "good" form of cholesterol linked to reduced rates of heart disease, HDL, and in fact soy protein has been reported in some studies to even increase HDL levels. Individuals who consume 20 to 30 grams of soy protein daily have been reported to lower their total cholesterol by 10 mg/dl on average. The higher one's cholesterol to begin with, the more significant the decrease when soy products are added to the diet.

Soy containing foods also are a good source of many vitamins such as folate and minerals such as iron. Soy is thought to have a beneficial effect on amino acids and proteins in the body as well as contribute isoflavones (genistein and daidzein) and phytoestrogens. Women who desire an "estrogen effect" without taking estrogens have flocked to soy as an excellent source of natural estrogens. Studies have been mixed regarding the beneficial effect of these phytoestrogens on bone, heart, and general well being and questions remain regarding their risk in women with breast cancer. Women who are dealing with problematic menopausal symptoms without a history of breast cancer may try phytoestrogens as an alternative to short term estrogen use.

The FDA and the American Heart Association has recommended that people consume 25 grams of soy protein per day as part of a diet low in saturated fat and cholesterol to help lower elevated cholesterol levels. Of note, soy protein is different from most other proteins derived from vegetable sources and is considered to be a "complete" protein similar to animal proteins though more healthy. In other words, soy protein contains all of the essential amino acids in sufficient quantities necessary for proper health and functioning. Another benefit is that soy protein reportedly causes less calcium to be lost from the bones as compared to animal proteins. Soy is no longer only for Hippies and vegetarians and should be considered part of a healthy diet.

The following are some additional facts about soy:

Soy Fiber

There are three types of soy fiber: okara, soy bran, and soy isolate fiber. All are high quality, inexpensive sources of dietary fiber. Soy bran is made from the outer covering of the soybean, or hull. The hulls contain a fibrous material that can be extracted and refined for use as a food ingredient. Soy isolate fiber is soy protein isolate in a fibrous form.

Lecithin

Lecithin can be extracted from soybean oil and is used in food manufacturing as an emulsifier in products that are high in fats and oils. Lecithin promotes stabilization of food while preventing oxidation, crystallization, and spattering. Lecithin is also a precursor in the body that is used to produce acetylcholine, a neurotransmitter that is thought to be the major chemical in the brain responsible for our memory.

Soy Flour

Soy flour is made from roasted soybeans ground into a fine powder. Soy flour is 50% protein and a good source of protein when added to recipes. It can be obtained in a "defatted" or "full-fat" form. The defatted form has an even more concentrated source of protein of 70% and retains most of the bean's dietary fiber. Soy flour is gluten free. When used in the production of yeast-raised bread, it is said to have a more dense texture. Since soy flour is free of gluten, however, it fails to provide structure to yeast-raised breads. For this reason, soy flour cannot replace all of the wheat or rye flour in a bread recipe. Using 15% soy flour in a recipe, however, produces a dense bread that has a pleasant nutty flavor. Baked products that are not yeast-raised, such as "quick breads", can use soy flour for up to 1/4 of the total amount of the flour called for in the recipe. Soy flour can be used to thicken gravies and cream sauces or be used to make homemade soymilk. Full-fat soy flour should be stored in the refrigerator or freezer to preserve its freshness; defatted soy flour is more stable and can be stored non-refrigerated on the shelf.

Soy Protein Isolate

This is yet another available form of soy protein that contains 90% protein produced from defatted flakes. This is a highly digestible source of amino acids. While it has little flavor in itself, it can be used in almost any food. Soy protein isolate should be kept sealed and dry though remains stable for many months. It can be easily added to a variety of cereals, shakes, soups, sauces, among many other meals as it provides protein and other nutrients without affecting the flavor of the food to which it is added. It may also come in flavors that might enhance a shake.

Soy Protein, Textured

Textured soy protein refers to products made from textured soy flour and textured soy protein concentrate. Textured soy flour is produced by processing defatted soy flour or soy protein concentrate through an extrusion cooker in order to compress the product. It contains 50% protein as well as the dietary fiber and soluble carbohydrates found in the soybean. It has long been used as a low cost additive for meat as a way of extending portion size. It can be obtained in either a granular or chunk style. Textured soy protein also is available as a "concentrate" with 70% protein content and dietary fiber. It also comes dried and when hydrated, assumes a chewy texture that mixes well with other foods. One 12-ounce package of soy burger-style crumbles is equivalent to approximately one pound of ground beef in most recipes. Recently, a variety of flavors have been added to soy products to have them resemble the taste of beef, turkey, and even pork. Textured soy protein has a long shelf life. It will keep for several months if it is stored in a tightly closed container at room temperature. Once it has been rehydrated, however, it must be stored in the refrigerator and used within a few days. Textured soy protein will triple in volume when hydrated. For example, one pound of dry textured soy protein will make approximately 3 pounds of hydrated textured soy protein. For recipes calling for one pound of ground beef, you can substitute 1 1/2 cups of dry textured soy protein and hydrate it with 1 1/2 cups water.

Soybean Oil

Soybean oil is also known as soyoil and is the natural oil extracted from whole soybeans. It is the most widely used oil in the US accounting for more than 75% of the total vegetable oil used. Oil sold commonly as "vegetable oil" is usually 100% soybean oil or a blend of soyoil and other oils. Soyoil is cholesterol free and high in polyunsaturated fat (61%) and monounsaturated fat (24%) and an excellent source of Vitamin E. It is frequently used in making margarines. Soybean oil is a good natural source of both linoleic and linolenic acids, both essential to humans. More than 50% of the fat in soy is linoleic acid; 7% of the fat is linolenic.

Soynut Butter

Soynut butter is made from roasted, whole soynuts which are crushed and blended with soybean oil and other ingredients. Soynut butter has a mild, nutty taste, contains less fat than peanut butter, and has a nutritionally sound profile.

Green Vegetable Soybeans (Edamame)

Commonly eaten in Japanese restaurants, these large soybeans are harvested at 80% maturity when the beans are still green and have a sweet taste. They can be eaten as either a snack or as part of a meal. They are either steamed or prepared by boiling in slightly salted water for 15 to 20 minutes. They are high in protein and fiber, contain no cholesterol and are a tasty treat. They are also available frozen both in the pod and shelled. Restaurants may add salt to the edamame and it may be beneficial to request that they defer this process if you are trying to limit your salt intake.

Do not eat soybeans raw. Soybeans must be cooked to destroy the protease inhibitor that is contained within the beans. Heating is necessary to deactivate this activity and make the beans digestible.

When cooking yellow soybeans, do not add salt or acidic ingredients, such as lemon juice, vinegar, or tomatoes until the beans are thoroughly cooked. Acidic additives delay the softening process. Black soybeans are an exception and in fact, acidic additives may help this form of soybean retain its shape through the cooking process.

When cooking dry soybeans, it is important to first soak the soybeans in 4 cups of water for each cup of beans for 8 hours. If you plan on soaking any longer than this time, make sure you refrigerate the beans. Drain and rinse the beans, add 4 cups of fresh water for each cup of beans you started with, and bring to a boil. Once boiling, reduce the heat, skim off any "foam" that has developed, and simmer for approximately 3 hours being careful to add more water as necessary. Cook until the beans are tender. One cup of dry beans will yield approximately 2–3 cups of cooked beans.

Miso

Miso is a rich, salty food that can be used to make miso soup or to flavor a variety of foods such as soups, sauces, salad dressings, marinades and even pates. Miso is a smooth paste that is made from soybeans and a grain such as rice. To this mixture, the manufacturer adds salt and a mold culture prior to "aging" in cedar vats for long periods of time, usually between one and three years. Miso paste requires refrigeration.

Natto

Natto is a fermented, cooked dish consisting of whole soybeans. The fermentation process degrades the beans' complex proteins and therefore is considered to be more easily digested than whole soybeans. It has a sticky viscous coating that has a cheese-like appearance. Traditionally, natto is used as a topping for rice, added to miso soups, or used with vegetables.

Okara

Okara is a pulp fiber by-product of soymilk. While it has less protein than whole soybeans, the protein is of high quality. Its taste is similar to coconut and it can be baked or added as fiber to granola or baked goods. A sausage has also been made from okara.

Soybeans

As with other beans, soybeans undergo a maturation process from the early green phase to a ripened form that is hardened and dry. There are several varieties of soybeans including the yellow, brown and black variety. Whole soybeans can be soaked and then roasted and eaten as a snack food. They do require cooking of some form though the green-yellow bean is most commonly boiled or steamed prior to serving (see Edamame).

Soymilk

Soybeans that are soaked, ground fine and strained produce a fluid that has been called soybean milk or soymilk. It is lactose- and casein-free and is available in regular and low-fat varieties. Some brands are fortified with calcium, Vitamin D, and/or Vitamin B12. Soymilk can be found in a variety of flavors including plain, vanilla, egg nog, chocolate, and even strawberry. Soymilk has gained a great deal of favor as a substitute to cow's milk due to it being well tolerated, especially for those who are lactase deficient. Milk sugar or lactose requires an enzyme in the intestine (lactase) to be broken down and absorbed. If this process does not occur, the milk sugar serves as an osmotic that produces loose bowl movements, gas and indigestion. Lactase deficiency is quite wide-spread with a higher percentage of African–Americans and elderly persons effected. The lactase enzyme may also be reduced at any time in one's life by intestinal illness even in individuals who once had normal enzyme levels. Plain, unfortified soymilk is an excellent source of high-quality protein and B vitamins. Most commercially produced brands have added calcium in a similar concentration as that found in cow milk, or approximately 300 mg calcium in every 8 ounce glass. The consumer is advised to read the label to determine the exact amount of calcium and other nutrients that have been added.

Soynuts

Soynuts are usually roasted and are made from whole soybeans that have been soaked in water and then baked until brown. They are often "flavored" and may even be sold covered in chocolate. They are high in protein and isoflavones and have a similar texture and flavor to peanuts.

Soy Sauce

Soy sauce is a dark liquid that is made from soybeans that have been fermented. It generally has a salty taste and sodium but can also be obtained in a "low salt" variety with approximately 1/3 less salt. Soy sauce can be found in three types, shoyu, tamari, and teriyaki. Shoyu is a blend of soybeans and wheat; tamari is made only from soybeans and is a by-product of making miso; teriyaki sauce is thicker and includes other ingredients like sugar, vinegar, and certain spices. Soy sauce is used to enhance the flavor of certain foods, such as fish though it is also gaining acceptance as a salad dressing and marinade.

Sprouts

Soybean sprouts are an excellent source of protein and Vitamin C and can be used in a similar fashion as other sprouts, such as mung bean sprouts or alfalfa spouts.

Tempeh

Tempeh is a traditional food from Indonesia. It is a chunky, tender soybean cake that is made from whole soybeans that are usually mixed with another grain such as rice or millet. This mixture is allowed to ferment and forms a rich cake of soybeans that has a nutty or smoky flavor. Tempeh can be marinated and grilled. It can also be cut into smaller squares and added to soups or casseroles.

Tofu

Tofu or soybean curd is a soft cheese-like food that is made by curdling fresh hot soymilk with a coagulant. It is a favorite of cooks because of its lack of flavor and ability to take on the flavor of the dish it is added to or the marinade it is placed into. Tofu is rich in high-quality protein and B vitamins and low in sodium. It comes in a variety of forms. Water-packed tofu (firm or extra firm) is a dense solid that can be easily cut into smaller portions and added to soups or stir-fry dishes. It can also be grilled and eaten as the main protein source of a meal. It is also higher in protein and calcium than the other forms of tofu. The water must be squeezed out prior to cooking to help maintain its form.

Soft tofu is best used in recipes that call for it to be blended into the meal. Silken tofu is a creamy, custard-like product that can be used to replace sour cream in blended or pureed dishes. It also makes an excellent foundation for "dips".

Yuba

Yuba is made by skimming and then drying the thin layer formed on the surface of hot soymilk as it is allowed to cool. Yuba has a high protein content and is sold in one of three forms, fresh, half-dried, or as dried bean curd sheets. The latter are often used in place of noodles in stir-fry dishes, casseroles, and even soups.

Garlic

Garlic has been considered a very special food since ancient times. It was worshipped by the ancient Egyptians and used by Greek athletes to enhance performance. Europeans of old wore garlic as necklaces in an attempt to ward off vampires and even as late as the early 20th century, it was thought to help one avoid contracting polio. In the latter case, it most likely worked by discouraging contact from others due to its potent odor. Although the data is not always convincing, garlic has been used to help fight against harmful bacteria, reduce cholesterol and heart disease, improve impotence, and even fight cancer.

There are over 12 worldwide studies confirming that garlic intake helps reduce blood cholesterol levels by as much as 12%. Levels of triglycerides have also been shown to be reduced by approximately 17% in persons taking garlic as compared to placebo. Garlic's antimicrobial powers were first identified by Louis Pasteur who acknowledged that garlic was as effective as penicillin in killing bacteria in test tubes. More recent data has also favorably compared its *in vitro* (in test tubes and not in humans) powers to the more potent antibiotic chloramphenicol. While highly debatable and not supported by well-designed clinical studies, garlic was historically used to treat infections caused by *Mycobacterium tuberculosis*, the organism responsible for causing tuberculosis or TB. While folklore stated it worked because of the sulphur compounds it contains, there is no evidence for its use as an anti-microbial at this time.

Folklore has also claimed that garlic has a potent aphrodisiac effect. Recent data suggests that garlic is capable of stimulating the production of nitric oxide synthase, an enzyme responsible for producing nitric oxide, the major mediator of erections. While still conjectural, it does provide food for thought!

While many have claimed that garlic can boost the immune system, it may also have an effect on cancer. Experimental studies have demonstrated that certain compounds found in high concentration in garlic have certain anti-tumor effects in the laboratory. One such compound, diallyl disulphide, reportedly reduced tumor growth by 50% when injected into tumors experimentally grown in animals. Another compound found in garlic, S-allylcysteine, reportedly prevents cancer causing agents from binding to human breast cells. No clinical data are yet available to demonstrate a direct effect of garlic on reducing levels of cancer in humans. While additional data are clearly needed to help us appreciate all of the potential benefits from garlic, for now, garlic remains a food that provides interesting flavor and perhaps benefit for our bodies!

Phytoestrogens

Phytoestrogens are plant compounds that are converted to estrogen like substances in the intestine. The most common source for these in the human diet are in the form of isoflavones that come mostly from soybeans. Tofu, a processed form of soy, contains less than the beans themselves. Lignans, present in high concentrations in flaxseed are also present in certain cereals, fruits, and vegetables. Black cohosh is also thought to have estrogenic properties derived from triterpenoid glycosides and isoflavones contained within. Red clover, another source of estrogenic activity, contains coumestrol, an isoflavone also found in soybeans.

Phytoestrogens act as weak estrogens, though in certain circumstances, as with the case of lignans, may bind to estrogen receptor sites and actually have an anti-estrogenic effect. These effects most commonly have been described as effecting uterine and vaginal cells though if taken in excess, they could interfere with hormone replacement therapy.

While still controversial, data suggests that phytoestrogens may have effects similar to estrogen used medicinally. Asian women consuming higher amounts of soy in their diet reportedly have fewer hot flushes at the time of menopause. Soy intake has been linked epidemiologically with a lower incidence of breast cancer in at least one study though this is in contrast to popular thinking that any form of estrogen may stimulate breast cancer growth and is deserving of additional study.

Of note, a randomized study in 104 post-menopausal women demonstrated that the addition of soy protein to the diet reduced symptoms of hot flushes. Another controlled study of 145 post-menopausal women reported that the addition of soy containing foods and flaxseed in the diet for 12 weeks reduced the number of hot flushes and vaginal dryness compared to control subjects; no difference was noted, however, in overall menopausal symptoms. A double-blind six-week crossover study in 51 post-menopausal women reported that 20 grams of soy protein added to the diet resulted in a reduction in the severity of menopausal symptoms. While one study did report an increase in breast cell proliferation in premenopausal women using large amounts of soy, no definitive adverse clinical findings have been reported to date. Women who already have a history of breast cancer may want to discuss this with their physicians prior to increasing their intake of any phytoestrogen containing food source. For now, soy based products remain an excellent source of vegetable protein and may offer some benefits to women seeking an alternative to hormonal replacement therapy. Other benefits from this weak form of estrogen have not been clearly delineated though are possible. Soy in the diet may reduce serum cholesterol concentrations, though clinical benefit has not been demonstrated in this regard.

Hemp

To many, the word "hemp" is synonymous with the 1960's and has a negative connotation. While it is true that hemp comes from the same plant species as marijuana, that is where the similarity ends. Hemp seeds are rich in protein and are a potent source of essential fatty acids, Vitamin E, and other antioxidants. Even though hemp seeds contain little to no THC, the psychoactive component of marijuana, the US Drug Enforcement Agency or DEA has attempted to ban the use of hemp in any form and especially in food. While the debate rages in the US Circuit Court of Appeals as to the constitutionality of such a ban, hemp foods can be legally imported, sold, and eaten.

Hemp seeds have found their way into granola, natural health bars, and even frozen waffles. Hemp oil is sold for salad dressing and hemp seeds can be eaten plain or sprinkled over salads or other foods.

A particular benefit from consuming hemp oil and seeds is its high content of essential fatty acids. These are necessary for proper functioning of the brain, heart and other body organs. Since your body does not make these, we are dependent on dietary sources. Fortunately, they are also bountiful in many other suggested foods such as flaxseeds, spinach, walnuts, and salmon. Hemp seeds also provide gamma-linolenic acid or GLA. This is an omega-6 fatty acid that is thought to have a beneficial effect on blood pressure. Some have suggested that it can have a positive effect on skin conditions such as eczema. Clearly not all of the data is in yet, though hemp may very soon turn out to be just what the doctor ordered.

Walnuts

<u>One Ounce, approximately 14 walnuts</u>
Calories: 190
Protein: 4 grams
Carbohydrate: 4 grams
Total Fat: 17 grams
Saturated Fat: 1.5 grams
Monounsaturated Fat: 2.5 grams
Polyunsaturated Fat: 13 grams
Linoleic Acid: 10.78 grams
Linolenic Acid: 2.57 grams
Cholesterol: 0 milligrams
Fiber: 2 grams

Significant amounts of manganese, copper, zinc, potassium, phosphorus, magnesium, iron, and calcium.

Walnuts have been enjoyed for thousands of years throughout the world. In fact, excavations in the southwest region of France have uncovered petrified shells of nuts that were roasted during the Neolithic period, more than eight thousand years ago. Walnut groves were painted on cave walls as far back as 2000 B.C. and were thought to exist within Mesopotamia in the famous Hanging Gardens of Babylon. Ancient mythology tells the story of a young woman being transformed into a walnut after death by Dionysus. The goddess Artemis carried this message to her father and ordered that a temple be built in her memory. The temple's columns were carved in wood in the form of young women and were called catyatides, or nymphs of the walnut tree.

The name of the walnut tree and its nut is formally known as Juglans regia (walnut tree) and nux juglandes (the walnut) derived from the expression "royal nut of Jove". The word "nut" is itself derived from the Latin name for nucleus, or fruit of the shell. Some believe it also was named for the Latin word night, or "nox" due to the dark juice of the nut which was used to dye wool in ancient times.

The walnut and its oil has been used for centuries and cherished as a valuable and health promoting food. The first commercial planting of the walnut tree in the US is thought to date to 1867 when Joseph Sexton planted English walnuts in Santa Barbara County, California. The Central Valley of California is considered to be the prime walnut growing region in the US due to ideal climate and fertile soils. California walnuts account for 99% of the commercial supply in the US and approximately 70% of the world's supply.

What makes the walnut so unique is not only its taste that has been enjoyed in a variety of foods, desserts, and as a snack for generations, but more recent data that has demonstrated a beneficial effect in reducing the risk of heart disease. In fact, the US FDA has issued a report stating that "supportive but not conclusive research shows that eating 1.5 ounces of walnuts as part of a diet low in saturated fat and cholesterol may reduce the risk of heart disease." This amount of walnuts contains approximately 2.5 grams of omega-3 fatty acid, almost ten times that found in almonds, the second best source.

Epidemiologically, data suggests that populations that consume nuts and walnuts in particular have a lower cardiovascular risk. This is largely thought to result from the high concentrations of omega-3 fatty acids present in nuts and particularly high in walnuts.

One and one-half ounces of walnuts provides the daily requirement of essential omega-3 fatty acids. Walnuts contain a myriad of other valuable vitamins, minerals, protein, and antioxidants. Next to rose hips, walnuts are the largest single source of antioxidants per gram. Omega-3 fatty acids have been shown to reduce inflammation and prevent aggregation of platelets, a process thought to be of prime importance in causing heart attacks. Omega-3 fatty acid ingestion has been shown to reduce C-reactive protein (CRP) in the body, a marker of dangerous inflammatory processes that have been linked to coronary artery disease.

Walnuts also contain a significant amount of the gamma-tocopherol form of Vitamin E, thought to promote an uptake of alpha-tocopherol into cells so that it can serve as a potent anti-oxidant and protect cells from oxidation damage.

Almonds

<u>One Ounce</u>
Calories: 164
Protein: 6 grams
Carbohydrate: 5.6 grams
Fat: 14.4 grams
Fiber: 3.3 grams
Calcium: 70 milligrams
Magnesium: 78 milligrams
Selenium: 2.2 micrograms
Phosphorus: 134 milligrams
Alpha-tocopherol (Vitamin E): 7.4 milligrams.

Almonds have long been sought as exotic treats and sources of nutrition. The Vikings would bring their bounty of almonds from afar and claim victory over foreign lands. Perhaps this is why the Scandinavians found creative ways to incorporate these treasures into the diet, especially in the form of marzipan, a mixture of finely ground almonds and sugar. Almonds have also been enjoyed for centuries either plain, made into a "butter", or used in cooking. A recent study reported that almonds may offer a lot more than just culinary pleasure. Individuals were randomly assigned to one of two diet groups with both groups consuming the same number of daily calories over a six month period of time. The group that lost more weight (18% versus 11%), had a greater drop in waist circumference (14% versus 9%), and had a larger reduction in blood pressure (11% versus 0%) had a greater percentage of their calories derived from fat (39% versus 18%) with the majority of the fat in the form of monounsaturated fat. This group ate a daily three-ounce portion of almonds. The authors concluded that adding almonds to a long-term low-calorie diet enhanced weight loss and significantly improved risk factors associated with heart disease. While the study also demonstrated that individuals in both diet groups had lower glucose and insulin levels at the conclusion of the study, medication requirements for individuals with type 2 diabetes decreased more significantly in the group that ate the low-calorie, almond supplemented diet as compared to the other diet with similar calories but without almonds. This study confirmed that not all calories are equivalent in terms of their effect on the body and health and that almonds may have a beneficial effect beyond their taste.

One possible explanation for the findings is that the fat in almonds may not have been completely absorbed; this would result in fewer available calories for the body to metabolize. This would be completely compatible with an older study that demonstrated that cell walls of almonds are capable of acting as a physical barrier to the absorption of fat and thus cause the body to excrete a higher percentage than otherwise would occur. Almonds, even in small, one ounce quantities, have been reported to provide a "full" and satisfied feeling, also helping to reduce one's appetite despite the lower calorie intake.

Almonds have been associated with improved lipid profiles and reduced low density lipoprotein levels (LDL-cholesterol) that has been linked to heart disease. In fact, LDL cholesterol was reduced by 35% with a diet containing almonds, oatmeal and other foods rich in viscous fiber, plant sterol-enriched margarine and foods high in soy protein; this effect was similar to that induced by cholesterol lowering drugs such as statins.

The FDA recently approved the first qualified health claim supporting the use of nuts in the diet. Their report states that "one and a half ounces of most nuts, including almonds, may reduce the risk of heart disease when they are part of a diet low in saturated fat and cholesterol". Clearly, every little addition to the diet that may have proven benefit will work in concert with other beneficial nutrients to promote greater health and well-being.

Flaxseeds

<u>One Tablespoon, approximately 1/3 ounce</u>
Calories: 59
Protein: 2.3 grams
Carbohydrate: 4.1 grams
Total Fat: 4.1 grams
Fiber: 3.3 grams.

Flaxseeds have been eaten for centuries as a laxative and as a "healthy" component of cereals and breads. Known as linseed in Europe, they have grown in popularity since it became known that they are an excellent source of omega-3 fatty acids. They also contain lignans, a type of fiber that is thought to have antioxidant properties and phytoestrogens. Lignans are broken down by bacteria in the digestive tract and converted into estrogen-like substances called enterodiol and enterolactone. While these substances are labeled estrogen-like, they bind to the estrogen receptor and at least in some studies, they have been demonstrated to exert a beneficial effect on estrogen sensitive breast cancer perhaps by interfering with the binding of endogenous estrogens. Also flaxseed oil lacks lignans in its natural form but may have them added in commercially available preparations.

These small, oval-shaped seeds come from the flax plant and are grown in abundance in several European countries including Belgium, France, Germany, and Russia. In the United States, they are primarily grown in Minnesota, Montana, North and South Dakota, and Texas.

The flax plant is very economical and is primarily grown as a source of linen, paper, linseed oil and flaxseed oil. Linseed oil plays a role in the production of paints, varnishes, and linoleum. The seeds can be used whole though they are better digested if ground prior to being added to food. They can be either added as part of the food preparation process or sprinkled over the food prior to serving. They are commonly added to cereals, breads, salads, casseroles, and desserts. Flaxseeds when combined with water and blended turn to a thick mixture that some recommend using instead of eggs in cooking recipes. Flax oil can be used as a salad oil though is unstable at high temperature and must not be used as a cooking oil. Flaxseeds themselves spoil easily if they are not stored in an airtight container and kept in the refrigerator, a process that can prolong their use for one to two months.

Flaxseeds have played a role in improving "digestion" for centuries. This most likely results from its "bulk-forming" qualities and use in preventing and treating constipation. Flaxseeds have a relatively high fiber content and also contain mucilage that allows it to expand when it comes in contact with water. This provides a stimulus to the bowels and more regular evacuation. Bulky bowel movements may also create a healthier environment in our intestines by reducing the pressure that the intestines normally need to eliminate their contents. This reduces the risk of developing diverticulae, or out-pouchings in the walls of the intestine; more regular bowel movements also reduce the time that potential toxins remain within the bowel and thus reduce the risk of colon cancer. Some have argued that a high bulk stool also serves to "cleanse" the bowl by removing small polyps and abnormal cells that may form.

Flaxseed is an excellent source of soluble fiber, linked to improved cholesterol. One study reported that individuals who consumed 20 grams of fiber per day in the form of defatted flaxseed had lower LDL-cholesterol levels. This study was of importance since the oil, a source of omega-3 oils, was first removed and thus any beneficial effect could not be considered due to these oils. Another study demonstrated that women who consumed 50 grams of raw flaxseeds per day for a month, or approximately 1.75 ounces, added to bread had a 9% decline in total cholesterol and an 18% decrease in LDL-cholesterol.

Flaxseeds contain alpha-linolenic acid, an omega-3 fatty acid and a precursor of EPA, a fatty acid found in fish oils. As mentioned previously, alpha-linolenic acid is an essential fatty acid and is important in cell membrane development and blood pressure regulation. While alpha-linolenic acid is converted to EPA in the body, and has beneficial effects on reducing LDL-cholesterol, it does not appear to lower triglyceride levels by itself. These fatty acids may also work to reduce blood clotting and thus lessen the chance of a heart attack. A study conducted in France in 1999 reported that a diet rich in alpha-linolenic acid, in this case being derived from a canola-oil margarine, significantly reduced the risk of developing a second heart attack in those with existing cardiovascular disease.

The lignans in flaxseed have also been reported to help alleviate menopausal symptoms including hot flashes, vaginal dryness and even memory impairment, though there is little scientific data to support these claims. Flaxseed contains more lignan precursors than any other plant food. Lignans are produced in the intestines by bacteria that convert the flax precursors into different lignan molecules that may more readily enter the bloodstream.

Lignans reportedly compete with estrogen for binding to its receptors and have also been shown in animal studies to be anti-angiogenic, or capable of limiting vessel growth in tumors. Human breast cancer cells implanted into immune deficient mice were less able to multiply if mice were fed flaxseeds. These animals additionally had a down-regulation of insulin like growth factor 1 (IGF-1) and epidermal growth factor in the cancer cells. Another study reported a down-regulation of the Her2 receptor in breast cancer cells of mice fed with flaxseed. Women newly diagnosed with breast cancer who were given a daily single muffin containing 25 grams of ground flax seeds as compared to control subjects given a wheat muffin without flax were reported to have a signifiant reduction in the expression of the cancer growth receptor Her2 and an increase in the apoptosis index of their breast cancer cells. Women waiting surgery for breast cancer who ate a flaxseed muffin daily containing approximately four tablespoons of ground flaxseeds reportedly had a slower tumor growth rate.

A study of 25 men with prostate cancer demonstrated that those who ate one ounce of ground flaxseeds, or approximately three tablespoons daily as part of a very low fat diet, were able to slow the progression of their cancers between the time of diagnosis and surgery as compared to those men who did not consume flaxseeds. Laboratory studies in rats show that lignans may slow the growth of colon tumor cells and reduce abnormal cell growth, an early marker for the development of colon cancer. It appears that the actual dose of lignans consumed may play a role. Additional research is clearly needed to better determine if there is any risk to taking flaxseeds in large quantities and what dose may prove beneficial as well as to confirm the above reported findings in larger, well controlled clinical trials.

There is also a body of literature that suggests that flaxseeds may have a beneficial effect on the kidney in persons with lupus, a connective tissue disease that frequently leads to kidney failure and inflammation. This is thought to be due to the high anti-oxidant effect of flaxseeds. Studies have also reported a possible association between Crohn's disease and low levels of omega-3 fatty acids. Animal data suggest that alpha-linolenic acid supplementation in the diet helps reduce bowel inflammation in an experimental model. Several studies have also suggested that omega-3 fatty acids are capable of reducing symptoms of rheumatoid arthritis including joint tenderness, morning stiffness, reduced mobility, and use of pain medication. Omega-3 fatty acids have also been used with some reported success for treating depression, burns, acne, asthma, and even menstrual pain. For example, a Danish study of 200 women reported that those with the highest dietary intake of omega-3 fatty acids had the mildest symptoms associated with menstruation.

While claims have also been made that these fatty acids may be useful in the treatment of ulcers, migraine headaches, attention deficit/hyperactivity disorder, emphysema, psoriasis, glaucoma, Lyme disease and even panic attacks, no conclusive data are available upon which to base any definitive conclusions.

In addition, some have argued that while smaller doses may be helpful in combating illness, high doses are not without risk. Animal data suggest that high doses of lignans contained within flaxseeds can actually promote certain cancer cell growth; alpha-linolenic acid when found in high concentrations in the blood has been linked to a possible increased risk of developing prostate cancer. While high doses of alpha-linolenic acid have been reported to increase the risk of developing macular degeneration, studies have found that individuals with regular consumption of fish containing high levels of omega-3 fatty acids have a lower risk of developing this leading cause of blindness in the elderly.

Prior to using large quantities of flaxseeds or flaxseed oil, it is important to check with one's physician and to weigh all options. In addition, omega-3 fatty acids may increase the blood-thinning effects of aspirin or warfarin used as an anti-coagulant. While this effect may be useful at times, the dose of warfarin may need to be adjusted to prevent bleeding if flaxseeds are to be continued at their prior level. There have been reports of flaxseed use slowing the absorption of certain medications; caution is advised if taking flaxseeds at the same time as other medications if problems arise.

Sesame Seeds

Dried, 1 tablespoon
Calories: 52
Protein: 1.6 grams
Carbohydrate: 2.1 grams
Fat: 4.5 grams
Fiber: 1.1 gram

Roasted/toasted, 1 ounce
Calories: 160
Protein: 4.8 grams
Carbohydrate: 7.3 grams
Fat: 13.6 grams
Fiber: 4.0 grams

Sesame oil, 1 teaspoon
Calories: 45
Fat: 5 grams

Sesame paste, 1 tablespoon
Calories: 95
Protein: 2.9 grams
Carbohydrate: 4.1 grams
Fat: 8.1 grams
Fiber: 0.9 grams

Sesame seeds date back to the Assyrians who reportedly used them over 3,000 years ago. In China they were grown as a taste sensation for at least 2,000 years. The Egyptians used sesame seeds as a form of medicine and the Turks were reported to use sesame oil as far back as 900 B.C. Sesame seeds were brought to Europe from India during the first century and were used as a substitute for olive oil in certain regions. It reached the United States in the 17th century from Africa when it was brought by slaves who called it "benne".

All children are taught the familiar phrase "Open Sesame", a phrase that has its roots in the stories of the Arabian Nights. This refers to the "sudden popping" sound made when mature sesame seed pods split open. Over the years, sesame seeds have been used to treat anemia, blurred vision, and constipation. They have also been used for beauty oils and in cosmetics.

Sesame seeds have a nut-like flavor and can be used raw, ground, or toasted. Sesame seeds can be added to foods whole or sprinkled over vegetables, pasta, or casseroles. They can be ground and blended with butter or mayonnaise and used as a spread. Middle Eastern and Asian recipes use sesame seeds to make tasty marinades and dipping sauces as well as Halva and hummus.

The sesame seed is from the *Sesamum indicum* plant of the pedaliaceae family. This plant in different parts of the world is also known as benne, sim sim, and abongra. The plant is an erect tropical plant and grows to a height of 6 feet. Drought resistant, this plant has oblong leaves and white to light rose flowers. Each fruit is a grooved capsule that often contains in excess of 100 seeds.

The sesame seed contains approximately 55% of its weight as oil, and has a high concentration of antioxidants. Sesame seeds are in demand all over the world with most crops grown in China, India, and the West Indies. In the United States, they are grown in greatest quantities in the southern and western states. While the white seeds are most commonly sold in the US, other forms such as black, brown and red seeds are available.

CHAPTER

16

Foods for Specific Goals

Although many of the following foods have not been 100% proven to improve specific health measures by randomized controlled clinical trials, each contains nutrients that have been linked to health and may prove beneficial if incorporated into a well balanced and carefully chosen diet.

Foods that May Improve Our Vision

Spinach, broccoli, chard, collards, and kale (green vegetables): Data suggests that these foods contain a relatively high content of lutein, a substance that may help filter out rays that may harm the eye, particularly the macula, the area of the eye that allows us to see fine details and that deteriorates most commonly in older persons and those exposed to excessive amounts of UV light.

Carrots, peaches, pumpkins and persimmons (orange fruits and vegetables): These contain Vitamin A that is necessary for proper night vision.

Corn: Relatively high in zeaxanthin, corn is thought capable of promoting eye health throughout life.

Cold water fish (salmon, sardines, mackerel, and tuna): These fish contain high concentrations of omega-oils that are thought to be protective against age related damage to the retina.

Foods that May Improve Our Cardiovascular Health

Garlic: Studies have shown garlic capable of lowering cholesterol levels.

Onions: Studies have demonstrated beneficial effects on preventing platelet aggregation predisposing to heart attacks.

Dark chocolate: Studies have demonstrated positive effects on anti-inflammatory markers and also on preventing platelet aggregation, both key in preventing cardiovascular disease from developing and progressing.

Oats: These grains contain flavonoids and have been shown to reduce cholesterol levels.

Red wine and red grape juice: Long thought to help promote cardiovascular health when taken in moderation due to resveratrol, an antioxidant, in the grape's skin.

Cold water fish (salmon, mackeral, sardines, tuna): Omega oils have been shown to promote cardiovascular health.

Green tea: Studies conducted in Japan have demonstrated lower cholesterol in persons who drink at least 5 cups of green tea daily. Note that the Japanese tea cup is significantly smaller than that used in America and Europe though green tea comes in various brands and depending on how it is made, yields varying quantities of the beneficial chemicals necessary for health.

Blueberries, raspberries and blackberries: These berries contain relatively high concentrations of bioflavonoids that have proven benefit for our cardiovascular system by reducing inflammation and preventing platelet aggregation.

Pomegranate: May lower blood pressure and contains high concentrations of antioxidants.

Foods that May Have Beneficial Effects on Memory

Green Tea: Bioflavonoids are found in high quantities in tea, especially green tea. These may have beneficial effects on promoting memory.

Dark skinned fruits (red apples, nectarines, and grapes): These foods contain significant amounts of flavonoids in their skin and may promote health.

Foods That May Reduce Risk of Cancer

Garlic: Although controversial, garlic contains allyl sulfur, a compound that in animals retards cancer growth. No data in humans exists to conclude whether this is beneficial for sure.

Carrots, broccoli, pumpkin, and cabbage: Various studies have suggested at least some benefit in terms of cancer prevention though no definitive studies have been done to date upon which to make a final conclusion. While these foods contain relatively high quantities of Vitamin A and lutein, antioxidants that may help protect against cellular damage including cancer, some studies have actually liked the intake of high doses of Vitamin A with the development of certain cancers.

Red wine and/or red grape juice: The California Men's Health Study analyzed self-reported data from over 80,000 men aged 45 to 69. The risk of developing lung cancer was reduced by 2% with each glass of red wine consumed per month. Clearly alcohol has its own set of risk factors and the key here is moderation; non-alcohol containing red grape juice apparently has the same potential health benefit but may be relatively high in calories and sugar content depending on the source.

Blueberries, raspberries, blackberries, cranberries and other fruits and berries rich in anti-oxidants have been linked in some studies to reduced rates of certain cancers.

CHAPTER

17

The Mind-Body Connection and Its Role in Reducing Stress

Incorporating Mindfulness into Your Daily Life

It has long been known that there is a close connection between our state of mind and how we feel and function. Just look at the person suffering with depression. Not only may this result in a change in one's outlook and motivation, but depression may also impact one's ability to enjoy life's simple pleasures as well as affect our memory, appetite, and physiological functioning. We live in a hectic and busy world with many competing activities and demands on our personal lives. To many, this routine presents a challenge that is both invigorating and rewarding. Others, however, find their situation to be one filled with stress. Stress is part of everyday life and cannot be completely eliminated. It serves to stimulate us to respond to emergent situations and the unexpected. It has long been known that there are three aspects of stress, the stressor itself, one's individual perception of the stress, and the response, both physical and emotional, that the individual has to it. We are all affected differently by stress depending on our perceptions and ability to handle it. Individuals under stress, particularly from things that are out of their control, have a greater chance of developing hypertension, coronary artery disease, stomach ulcers, and other ailments. It has been noted that the greater the stressful situation or number of stressful situations that one must endure, the greater the chances of getting sick. Not all stress comes from negative events such as illness, the loss of a loved one, or some financial distress; stress can be associated with a life-changing positive experience as well. We all handle stress differently and the better prepared we are to deal with these everyday occurrences, the healthier we will be.

It is well known that stress results in a number of physiological responses known popularly as the "fight or flight" phenomenon. This response allowed us to run from enemies, escape from wild animals, and basically survive to live another day and procreate. The mediators of the stress response mostly come from our catecholamines, epinephrine and norepinephrine. These cause our heart and respiratory rates to increase; blood pressure to rise; blood to drain from the extremities and pool in the trunk and head; muscles tense; digestion slows; pupils become larger and thus our vision improves; hearing becomes more acute; and we have a feeling of increased strength, energy, and either aggressiveness or fear leading to flight.

Stressors come in many forms and can result from things that affect our body, mind, and environment. Examples of stress from the body include illness, injury, among others. The mind can cause us stress by providing us with worry, fear, and anxiety, whether due to real or just perceived feelings. The labels we put on various aspects of our life can lead us down different paths. The environment can create stress as well by way of producing changes in the weather, crowding, pollution, living situations, etc.

As noted above, stress can cause us to be ill and impact on our quality and even quantity of life. The following are common physical ailments that have been associated with stress: headaches, ulcers, heart disease, muscle tension, cancer, high blood pressure, spastic colitis, hyperventilation, insomnia, sexual dysfunction, stroke.

Emotional consequences of stress include: anxiety, worry, fear, guilt, anger, resentment, confusion, depression, helplessness and inadequacy.

Equally important, stress can result in changes in our behavior: irritability, compulsiveness, erratic behavior, hostility, loss of concentration, theft, complaints, and confrontation.

Stress may also lead to self-destructive behavior such as drug use, alcoholism, smoking, and eating disorders.

A number of years ago, Dr. Thomas Holmes attempted to quantitate the effects of stressful situations on one's health using actuarial data. Various stressors were rated as to their potential impact and each was assigned a specific number of "Life Changing Units". While there is a great deal of variation as to how a given stressor will affect any given individual, it is well worth noting that the effects of these stressors were shown to be accumulative. Eighty percent of individuals who had over 300 Life Changing Units, 50% of those with between 150 and 299 Units, and 30% of those exposed to less than 150 Units developed a major illness within the next two years.

The following listing from Dr. Holmes is available on the internet and attempts to quantitate "stressors":

Event	Units
Death of a Spouse	100
Divorce	73
Marital Separation or End of Love Relationship	65
Incarceration	63
Death of a Close Family Member	63
Personal Injury or Illness	53
Miscarriage or Abortion	53
Marriage	50
Fired at work	47
Retirement	45
Change in Health of a Family Member	44
Pregnancy	40
Birth of a Child	39
Change in Financial State	38
Mortgage above means	31
Change in Responsibilities at work	29
Child leaving home	29
Begin or End School	26
Change in Living Conditions	25
Trouble with Boss	23
Change in Work Hours or Conditions	20
Change in Sleeping Habits	15
Change in Eating Habits	15
Vacation	13
Christmas	12
Minor Violations of the Law	11

After marking off what individual stressors exist in someone's life, the assigned units are totaled and a risk assessment for developing major illness within the next two years can be calculated.

As mentioned above, a stressor is an event or situation in your life that results in a stress response. Stressors can be positive or negative with the most harmful ones being those that you perceive as having little control over. The truth is that in many cases you do have control at least in how you are able to handle the stress even if you do not have the power to eliminate it. Many everyday events are unavoidable and beyond your power to change. We often fail to recognize the warning signs that stress is building up and doing harm to our bodies and minds. Feeling excess stress can keep you from living a productive, happy, and healthy life; stress that is below the surface and not always apparent is equally as damaging.

A recent study reported that elderly persons are more vulnerable to stress. Using exposure to cold as a stressful stimulus, persons aged 18 to 33 and 65 to 89 were compared. After being subjected to their hand being placed in ice water, something that has been shown to raise cortisol levels, subjects were tested as to their ability to "drive" on a simulated track. Older subjects performed better than younger ones prior to being exposed to the stress. Following the stress, however, older subjects did worse with more braking, restarting and caution exhibited. Stress indeed did impact on the older person's decision-making ability more than on the younger person.

Stress is not the only example of the strong mind-body connection. Individuals who feel pessimistic or lack a positive attitude have been reported to have a harder time recovering from surgery. In fact, many surgeons postpone elective surgery until some form of psychological intervention can be done to bolster the patient's "will to suceed". Our outlook on life's events has powerful effects.

We also know from work done by Dr. Becca Levy, an Associate Professor of Psychology and Epidemiology at Yale University that individuals who were able to maintain a positive perception and attitude about their own aging process, live on average 7.5 years longer than those who do not. She also noted that individuals who were the subject of ridicule, referred to as "feeble", "forgetful", among other negative terms, performed significantly worse on tests that measured memory and balance as compared to similar individuals treated in a more respectful manner. Studies have also noted that elderly persons with dementia who were spoken to in an undignified manner were less likely to be cooperative or receptive to care and exhibited a greater amount of aggressive behavior, likely causing a greater degree of stress response and negative impact on health.

Many years ago while I was an Endocrine Fellow working in a hospital in Boston, I cared for patients in the Clinical Research Center who were either part of a clinical research study or were receiving individualized therapy that required careful monitoring and skilled nursing care thought best provided in that setting. It was there that I first met Herbert Benson, MD, Director of the Center and also the father of what became known as the Relaxation Response, the name of a book he wrote. In 1971, Dr. Benson and his co-authors were the first to publish a study on meditation titled "A Wakeful Hypometabolic Physiologic State"; this paper described a reduction in oxygen consumption during meditation. Dr. Benson has spent the past 30 years trying to foster beneficial relationships between the body and mind and has received a great deal of notoriety in doing so.

As previously mentioned, it is well known that our own bodies make certain substances popularly referred to as our "fight-flight" body chemicals or the catecholamines (epinephrine and norepinephrine) and cortisol. While these substances may help us in times of danger to increase our energy to fight off a foe or flee from danger, they also are capable of promoting illness. In fact, norepinephrine is a potent stimulator of "apoptosis" or programmed cell-death. Data has shown that persons with higher norepinephrine levels after a heart attack have greater myocardial cell damage and loss of viable heart tissue. For this reason among others, heart attack victims are usually treated with a medication known as a beta-blocker that prevents the catecholamines from exerting their effect at the cellular level.

Dr. Benson reported a link between high blood pressure and emotions and proved that we can indeed influence our blood pressure through a series of interventions that we can learn to do not only consciously but also subconsciously. While novel at that time, this concept has become well recognized and accepted as has the role of stress in promoting disease. In 1971, Dr. Benson and his co-workers published a paper that made major news when he reported that meditation was capable of reducing the amount of oxygen being used by 17%, lowering heart rates by as much as three beats a minutes, and increasing theta brain waves, those that immediately precede a sleep state.

Many persons have what is referred to as "white coat hypertension". This refers to a high blood pressure in the setting of a stressful situation such as going to the doctor; in a relaxed state, these same individuals have a normal blood pressure. Since treating such persons with anti-hypertensive medication may lead to too low a blood pressure most of the time, it has been suggested that no treatment is required for this form of stress induced hypertension. I have always taken exception to this; while I agree that medication may not be indicated and may result in unwanted side-effects, helping the effected person to be better able to "deal" with the stressful situation that leads to their body responding in such a potentially harmful manner is key and in itself deserves "treatment"! I have spent the last 30 years teaching this principle to both medical students and residents and discussing various ways that persons can be taught to better deal with stressful situations. Unfortunately, many persons in the medical profession only consider a medication as a treatment and thus do not even offer alternate therapeutic options.

It is also important to remember that stressful situations, perceived or subconscious, can lead to not only changes in blood pressure but other problems as delineated previously. Above I listed major "life-changing events" that may create varying amounts of stress. It is important to note, however, that many things not listed can be equally harmful. Most people lead hectic lives with numerous experiences, real or perceived, throughout the day that result in either conscious or sub-conscious stress. Whether it is waiting on a line at the supermarket, driving in congested traffic, dealing with a boss or work dead-line, waiting for a phone call, hearing news on the radio or TV, some financial problem, or some other daily occurrence, we need to be able to handle stressful situations in a manner that will not cause our body to increase its "fight-flight" hormones. We must all find ways to promote better insight, awareness, and inner calm!

I became increasingly intrigued with methods of inducing a "relaxed" state and realized early on that the better someone can handle their conscious and sub-conscious "stressors", the greater chance a person will have to lead a healthy and happy life. We now know that we do have the ability to control not only our emotions but also the way we "deal" with them in terms of our body's responses. When confronted with the same "stressor", no two persons respond in a similar manner. You have probably heard of a Type A versus a Type B personality. The Type A person is more "excitable", driven, and also prone to illness. While the Type B person may not achieve in the same way, they are likely better able to handle stressful situations with less wear and tear on their body. This does not mean that someone cannot be accomplished or still thrive in a high stress environment and be Type B, but rather, it is "how" we deal with the stress when it confronts us that will determine our health status over time.

I spent considerable time studying the endogenous opioid system, the endorphins, substances that are important regulators of pain and pleasure. It has been noted that these peptides, located in the brain, play a significant role in our appetite regulation, sexual pleasure, ability to withstand pain during situations such as childbirth, enjoyment in life's occurrences, and perhaps even addiction to exercise and other activities we participate in. Of note, studies have demonstrated higher endogenous opioid levels following certain forms of meditation.

We must all learn to recognize and gain a better understanding of what are the major stresses in our lives, both big and small, positive and negative. We need to appreciate the ways we currently "respond" to these stressful situations and lastly we must all learn to find ways to minimize stress and develop coping mechanisms during times when stress is unavoidable. Sometimes merely anticipating that an experience will lead to stress will allow one to avoid the situation completely; clearly, we cannot escape from all of life's stresses nor would it be a good thing to do so even if we could. You need to develop a lifestyle and environment as much as possible that allows you to function within your boundaries for dealing with stress. Being an air-traffic controller is not the profession of choice for all! Know your limits and strive for a balance between accepting challenges yet living within your limits of tolerance and ability to deal with the stress that may result from this choice of activity.

There are many ways to cope with stress. How well you are able to cope with unavoidable stress will clearly impact on your health. The following are several ways to help you be better prepared and promote a healthier you!

Try to avoid keeping frustrations to yourself. Seek the advice of family, friends, or members of the clergy or medical profession. Talking can help you identify a solution to a stressful situation.

Make sure that you obtain adequate sleep and eat a well balanced and nutritionally sound diet. Keep active as this is also an excellent way to alleviate stress. If you are able, "walk away" from the stresses of everyday life. This may involve taking a break to go outside, read, talk, listen to music, or take a moment to just be alone. Many persons become stressed from poor time management; this may lead to tasks not being able to be completed or poorly done. While it may not be possible to accomplish all that you set out to do in a given period of time, start by establishing goals for yourself and learn to set priorities. List those things you wish to accomplish with a realistic and attainable timeframe for doing so. Delineate both short and long term goals. Best of all, plan ahead to reduce the chances of something unexpected arising that may complicate your life.

Under certain circumstances, it may even be necessary to "walk away" completely from the stress producing situation — this should not be taken as a sign of failure or weakness but rather a life sustaining and health promoting change. This may involve changing jobs, leaving an abusive spouse, or other similar major alteration in one's life.

Practicing one of many methods to reduce your tension and stress on a regular basis will allow you to incorporate this coping mechanism into your subconscious, a powerful tool for helping you to handle stress and maintain your inner calm and health promoting state when necessary.

There are many ways to better manage one's own stress and each can be learned if there is the proper motivation to do so. The trick is to "internalize" the method so it becomes something that is done without thinking, much like our breathing.

One such method is meditation. While there are several ways to meditate, each with their own proponents, I am particularly drawn to the method of Mindfulness Meditation. Mindfulness refers to a meditation practice that fosters someone to be "present and aware" moment by moment, blocking out stress and distracting thoughts. When investigators measured brain waves in a group of Buddhist Monks who were doing Mindfulness Meditation and compared it to another group of skilled practitioners doing a form of Meditation that resulted in a deep trance, they reported a distinct difference. When a loud bell was sounded during the meditation, the deep Meditation practitioner's brain waves did not change as they were able to maintain the trance despite the noxious stimuli; those practicing Mindfulness Meditation, in contrast, kept in their state of meditation though their brain waves recorded activity in a similar manner to individuals who were told to directly focus on the sound and who were not even meditating. Despite the depth of the meditation, these monks were able to be aware and to notice things as they happened each and every moment, a lesson for us all. It is possible to be "present in the moment" and "aware" yet maintain calm and inner peace.

As mentioned above, Mindfulness is a meditation practice that focuses on the "present moment". It is not about thinking, interpreting, or evaluating a thought, event or person. It allows one to be present in a non-judgmental manner and allows one to be aware of what is happening continually yet to remain detached. It is not about anticipating or planning some future event or pondering something you have done or something from the past.

Any activity can be done with mindfulness and this technique can be practiced not only during prescribed times of meditation but while eating, exercising, talking on the phone, etc. Through this practice and finding ways to incorporate it into everyday life, you will have a greater degree of emotional equilibrium and well-being. This can be done throughout the day as you inwardly pause and become aware of your feelings and state. Although early on you will notice feelings such as happiness, sadness, nervousness, greed, anger, among other feelings and emotions, the more you practice Mindfullness in your everyday life, the easier time you will have learning to "let go" of these emotions and allow yourself to be more mindful of your own thoughts and actions.

During meditation practice, thoughts are allowed to come into the mind, but much like a host greeting guests at a party, the thoughts and/or emotions should be recorded and allowed to enter, but be escorted out of consciousness to be dealt with at a later time if one so chooses. While most people practice Mindfulness Meditation while seated in a specific posture to be described later, this form of meditation can be done while walking (Walking Meditation), sitting in a chair, or during some activity. This can also be extended to include Mindfulness to all areas of one's life. When I was younger, I particularly enjoyed watercolor painting as a way of practicing Mindfulness. Putting the paper on a counter, I observed the many colors and textures I had applied to my palette and with the stroke of a brush, "Mindfully" created images. While I have saved several of my paintings over the years, in the true spirit of Mindfulness, most of my creations were crumpled and discarded when my time to paint that day was over. I enjoyed the experience for what it offered at that moment, a calming and rejuvenating effect. No matter how talented someone is, in the privacy of one's own home it makes little difference and I suggest trying watercolor painting or perhaps some activity that you find enjoyable or challenging in a Mindful and accepting manner. After I had been practicing Mindful watercolor painting for a while, I noted my greater appreciation of the world around me such as the sounds of the birds, the sky's varied colors, the laughter of children. Everyone has to find their own path and what works for one person may not be appropriate for another. The trick is to find something, anything, and start!

Mindfulness Meditation is increasingly being recommended by health professionals as a way to control the pain of chronic illness including cancer and AIDS. It is being used to treat hypertension, depression, anxiety, and hyperactivity, among many other disorders. My son started his karate training at age 7 and by age 14 was a black belt, teaching as a Sensei in the after school program. I was always amazed when I would stop by the gym to see the 7 year olds in his karate class; despite the fact that just minutes before these young children were running and screaming and seemingly out of control, upon his request, they all assumed a meditation posture and remained still and attentive for what seemed like an eternity, though in reality for 10 to 15 minutes. How lucky these young children were to learn this technique so early in their lives; I only hope that they continued to practice and incorporate what they learned.

Meditation works to control stress and the better we are able to incorporate it into our lives, the greater the benefits we can achieve toward our overall health. Studies have provided evidence that meditation can help us re-program our minds. In other words, what was once a threshold for reacting to some stressful event, no longer elicits the same response; our brains have basically been reprogrammed and respond differently to the same stimulus.

Studies have shown that meditation blocks information from coming into the parietal area of the brain and reduces overall blood flow into the brain. Of note, individuals who meditate reportedly have increased blood flow into the limbic system, that part of the brain that is capable of generating emotions and memories and helps to regulate one's breathing, heart rate, and metabolism. Others have reported that meditation is capable of shifting brain wave activity from the right hemisphere to the left. This was felt to be a change from the typical "fight-flight" response areas of the brain to an area more associated with calming and acceptance. The left side of the brain is also thought to be more related to enthusiasm, relaxation, and happiness. Studies conducted using skilled meditators have shown a greater tendency of neurons to direct brainwaves to the frontal areas of the brain that relate to concentration. Mindfulness training has been used to modify behaviors with excellent results when used with incarcerated individuals. Rates of violence among inmates have been demonstrated to decline and the rate of return to prison reduced. It is particularly effective in helping to improve impulse control.

Perhaps one of the most well respected proponents of Mindfulness Training and Meditation is Dr. Jon Kabat-Zinn, founder of the Stress Reduction Clinic at the University of Massachusetts Medical Center in Worster, Massachusetts. Dr. Kabat-Zinn successfully helped teach persons suffering with chronic pain to manage with less or even no medication by teaching them to focus on their pain and "letting go" rather than "fighting it". He incorporated Mindfulness Training, meditation, and Body Scan Meditation to achieve his desired results. In a series of experiments, he additionally showed marked differences in the ability to resolve active psoriasis through the use of meditation and a higher antibody response following vaccination in those persons who practiced meditation as compared to control subjects who did not. These experiments demonstrated a relationship between the immune system and meditation.

The key to Mindfulness training is learning to "let go". Do not judge yourself or focus on what others say or think about you. Accept each and every moment "just as it is", not good or bad, but something to be enjoyed and accepted. Do not get distracted by thoughts, expectations, or goals. Through this, one can learn to be more accepting of self and others and be better able to handle stressful situations that may arise. Learn to love one-self and to accept who you are. We often are hard on ourselves and too often focus on what others think about us. While it is true that we can set goals for our own health and put ourselves on a proper path, there is no benefit to self-pity, anger, or frustration.

While meditation and mindfulness training are universal and not part of a specific religion or limited in its appeal and benefit, they were first adopted as a part of life many hundreds of years ago by the ancients in India and Japan. It was said that a practice that allowed someone to focus on the "present moment" would facilitate the release of suffering, something everyone was thought to witness at some time or another regardless of their status in life. "To live is to suffer" was the expression that prevailed. We will all be ill at some time in our lives; if we are fortunate enough, we will have problems that come with old age; we will see family and friends die. The list goes on and is very personal. How we choose and are able to deal with our own "suffering", however small or large it is, is something within our own grasp and worth considering before it becomes an overwhelming challenge.

Most practitioners of meditation have a method to allow their minds to "clear" or "let go". While some like to repeat a word or phrase, I have found the well accepted method of "counting breaths" to be most helpful. The following is a method that may work for you!

Dress comfortably in loose fitting clothing such as sweat pants and a Tee shirt.

Find a quiet place to "sit" that will allow you to remain without being disturbed for a period of time.

Make sure that the room temperature is appropriate, not too cold or warm.

Determine what type of posture you will assume; while most sit while meditating on the floor with straight back and crossed legs, a chair is also acceptable for those who find the floor too limiting or physically not possible. There are also various "stands" on the market that allow one to sit with knees bent behind them with less stress on the knee joints than would occur if one were to assume this posture without aid.

Meditation pillows can help facilitate one's proper posture and comfort to allow one to remain in the same position for a prolonged period of time without undue discomfort. The larger square or rectangular pillow is known as a zabuton and it provides the base upon which you will place a more firm and rounded pillow, the zafu. A carpeted floor is an equally good alternative for the zabuton. You should feel free to use any combination of pillows or cushions that will allow you to sit with legs crossed, either half or full "lotus", while maintaining a straight back. Many persons will not be able to sit in either the half or full "lotus" position due to discomfort, arthritis, or some other physical ailment. Do not let this discourage you from sitting while you meditate as any comfortable position that provides you with stability can be successful and is acceptable.

Experiment with what works for you! The idea of the zafu, or any smaller rounded pillow, is to allow you to angle yourself appropriately so that your body is like a solid mountain with your knees and behind being the points of contact and stability. You may need to experiment with pillows of varying firmness and height to achieve the "right" position for you.

However you sit, it is important to notice the stable nature of your posture as you focus your mind on the present moment. You should stretch first with your hands touching as far as they can to your left knee and then to the right. Your head is held high and erect as if there was a pulley to the ceiling. As you sit, you sway back and forth to the left and to the right, front and back until you find your proper place and "center". Your hands are placed at waist level with palms one over the other, left hand over right hand and the thumbs touching lightly. Let the tension leave your muscles starting at your feet and progressing to your head.

If you prefer to sit in a chair, make sure that it is the right height for you. Your knees should bend gently beneath you and a pillow on the floor to rest your feet may be useful to achieve the proper angle of your hips and knees. Sit on the front 1/3 of your chair and assume a straight posture with your hands at waist level similar to where they should be if you were sitting on the floor.

Your tongue is placed behind the upper front teeth and you rhythmically start to breath in and out. At first, focus on the breathing itself; be aware of the breaths, the sounds of your body and breath itself as it rhythmically creates its own focus. Then start to count on each out breath starting with 1 and going to 10. Slowly you concentrate as the breath comes in and goes out using your abdomen as a gauge for each respiration. In ... Out...Count to 10 and then start over again in a continuous relaxing and rhythmic manner. Breathe in to relax, calm, let go and breathe out to enjoy the moment and appreciate the oneness that has been created with your environment. As one becomes more experienced, the focus can be on the breathing alone without counting but there is no shame or difference if one must continue to count. If you find your counting going above 10, you were likely not paying attention; just start over again at 1 and you will be back on track. There is no harm in having to start again. This reflects the fact that your mind likely wandered off and needs to be gently returned to the path of mindfulness that you have begun.

Tilt your head somewhat downward, allowing your gaze to focus on a point two to three feet in front of you. Stare at that spot and allow your eyes to go out of focus as you continue your gaze. You are not to close your eyes as this will facilitate a sleep state and this is the farthest thing from your goal of full awareness and being in the moment.

Choose a time of the day that will "work" for you. It can be in the morning or later in the day but consistency is the best way to insure compliance. If possible, avoid practicing within two hours of eating to minimize the impact of the digestive processes on your efforts.

Start with 5–10 minutes and work up to 20–30 minutes at a sitting. Once or twice a week is a good start though you will likely want to increase the time and frequency of your "sitting periods" as you master the technique and appreciate the calming effect that it brings to you.

As you breath in, feel the "calm" that takes over your body; as you breath out, feel relaxed and at ease. Release any tension that you may have. Breathe in, relax; breathe out, release worry and anxiety and enjoy the moment you are in. You will soon accept that the present moment is a special one and you will appreciate being alive and fully aware.

Mindful breathing lets us be aware of our bodies and learn to accept it just as it is. Another technique is to recognize our body's parts as we breathe and "smile" to each and thus incorporate love and acceptance. This is particularly useful for those with physical ailments though learning to practice this when things are going well will help us to prepare for times when we may need to have this skill.

Experienced practitioners often combine "sitting meditation" with shorter periods of walking meditation, walking slowly at first keeping the rhythm of your breathing. This walking then shifts to a more rapid pace prior to resuming the sitting position and another period of sitting meditation. As you master this technique, Mindfulness will allow you to be one with the sounds, sights, tastes, and feelings of the world around you and to see things in a setting of greater compassion, joy, and understanding. You will not be limited to only these periods but learn to incorporate Mindfulness into each moment of the day regardless of your activity or situation.

I have found Mindful Meditation extremely useful in times of everyday stress. Some examples include being in traffic jams, having dental work performed, lying in an MRI machine, among many other stress provoking experiences. While the process of Mindful breathing will likely become second nature and something that you will find yourself doing even without thinking, even skilled practitioners may consciously decide that it is the "right" time to begin to count or focus on one's breaths as a way to return to the calm and relaxed state that we desire and need for lifelong health and happiness. Under certain circumstances, it may even be necessary to excuse oneself from a very stress provoking situation to allow one's stress to dissipate. As you master the technique, this may require only a few deep breaths or moments of Mindful Meditation while sitting or standing in a quite corner or perhaps walking outside or down a quite hallway. You will soon appreciate that certain methods work better for you than others and these techniques will soon become part of your everyday life to draw upon when necessary.

Mindful Eating

Practicing mindfulness during a meal is an excellent way to approach life, especially if you want to change your fast paced, hectic, and often mindless patterns. It is also an excellent way to begin to enjoy your meals more and help you master portion control and restraint. We often are not even aware of what crosses into our mouths, eating in a mindless and mechanical manner. How sad! Even before you start eating, pay close attention to what is before you. Look at each serving plate and notice the many colors, textures, and smells in anticipation of what is to come. When you put the food onto your own plate, once again pause before you start eating to activate all of your senses. Notice the variety of colors, shapes, textures, smells, and consistency of the food before you and then notice the taste of your food. As you place the food into your mouth, do it mindfully and slowly. Chew, swallow and hopefully digest each bite in a mindful manner, finishing each process before taking another bite into your mouth. Observe each food as you continue to eat, bite after bite much like the rhythm of your breath. Notice the taste of the food whether it is salty, sweet, sour, or bitter. Notice thoughts that come up in your mind and let them go. As you chew and begin to digest the food, notice the changing consistency of the food, often going from hard to soft or hot to cold.

It is important to stop at intervals during the meal. Perhaps a good time is when you drink mindfully from your beverage. Put down your knife and fork slowly and mindfully and pick up your glass, drinking slowly and deliberately. Notice what comes to mind as you let go of your thoughts and resume your eating.

When you are done eating, be mindful for a few moments, and breathe deeply, perhaps counting your breaths again from 1 to 10 on each outward breath.

You are now ready to resume your other activities in hopefully a more rested and mindful state! You will also find that this method helps control urges you may have to gorge on food in excessive quantities while also allowing your body to sense a full feeling and limit the amount of calories consumed to only those that are necessary and planned.

Relaxation Exercises

Another method that may help you to be better able to handle stressful situations is to consciously contrast moments of "tension" to states of "relaxation". In this way, your body will hopefully be able to understand differences in the way it responds and with experience, allow the subconscious to take over and set the stage for a more calm and relaxed you.

First, sit in a comfortable chair or lie on your back in a quiet location. Take a few deep breaths before resuming your customary and normal rhythmic breathing pattern. You will now begin to first tense and then release different groups of muscles, one at a time. Start with your hands. Make a fist and squeeze as tight as you can, first using the right hand. Notice the tension as you squeeze as hard as possible as you count to 5. Now, slowly lessen the grip to the count of 5 and notice the contrasting feeling. You feel relaxed and calm! Repeat this exercise three times and then do the same with the left hand.

Now move to your upper arm as you tense your right bicep as hard as you can and hold it to the count of 5. Repeat the same process that you did with your hand slowly releasing the tension and repeating this 3 times. Move to the other side and repeat.

This exercise should be repeated in a similar manner as you contrast tension and relaxation in your shoulders, eye-lids, mouth, toes, feet, calf muscles, thighs, and lastly the buttock muscles. You will notice the contrasting feelings between tension and relaxation, stress and calm.

By repeating this exercise on a regular basis, your body will learn to be able to better handle stressful situations. If your subconscious coping mechanisms fail to relieve the stress you are feeling on your own, you can start the process using the thigh muscles as this is something that can be done in almost any circumstance without alerting others to your process of stress reduction. Soon you will feel calm and relaxed again!

Body Scan Meditation

This form of meditation is best done when starting with a skilled practitioner either in person or on a tape/DVD guiding your movements. You can easily do this yourself once you master the routine. Lying flat on your back with your head on a pillow to create a soothing atmosphere, focus on a particular part of your body. Several methods may be used. The first teaches you to focus your awareness on a particular part of your body and to breathe deeply and rhythmically. As you inhale, breathe in awareness; as you exhale, release tension and any discomfort that may exist. The other method is to tense a particular part of your body and hold the tension to the count of 5 as you breathe slowly, counting on the "out" breath. You then release the tension and notice the calm, relaxed state of that part of your body. By starting at the head and working down to include all areas of the body, this Body Scan allows you to completely put yourself in a calm and aware state. Yet another method is to focus on each part of the body as you breathe in and out. With each "in" breath, feel relaxed and accepting of that body part; with each "out" breath, feel joy as you "smile" to that part of your body and appreciate it as being part of you!

This method of relaxation is harder to incorporate into your everyday experiences when challenged by a stressful situation. Nevertheless, any one of the above methods can be practiced daily as a way to promote relaxation and inner calm.

Bio-Feedback

Bio-Feedback requires special apparatus to help you to monitor your physical state while you attempt to control your physiological function using your mind. Whether you use breathing techniques, contrasting muscle tension/relaxation exercises, or some other method, these machines use a variety of measures to illustrate your success. One apparatus measures electrical impulses generated through the electrolytes in your sweat. It assumes that more tense individuals will give off more perspiration and thus you can see the moment to moment response as you attempt to establish calmness. Other machines measure blood pressure or heart rate. Once you master the technique, the subconscious takes over and you are better able to deal with stressful situations.

Centering or Concentrative Meditation

The method of "Centering" or "Concentrative" Meditation is said to allow you to have a relaxed yet still focused state of mind. This method is frequently used by athletes who are preparing for a race or competition. It is based on your own established method and therefore needs some trial and error prior to adopting a specific regimen. Only you will know when you have achieved your "Center" but returning to this state of calm will be something that you will be able to do freely and in any circumstance. Basically, this is a meditative technique that directs the mind to a single focus, such as the breath, a mantra, or image.

Examples of methods that may allow you to reach your "Center" include:

- Counting numbers up or down in rhythmic fashion.
- Repeating a phrase or word, perhaps a mantra, prayer, or poem.
- Repeatedly stretching various parts of the body in an orderly manner.
- Breathing deeply in and out.
- Counting breaths, in and out in a slow but rhythmic fashion.
- Writing a sentence or word over and over again focusing on the writing.
- Focusing on a sound to help bring you to a "Center" point in your body. This can be a continuous sound or one that occurs periodically over time, allowing you to re-center yourself continually.
- Focusing on a visual object and using that as a way of centering your mind.

Loving-Kindness Meditation

This form of meditation is intended to help one cultivate a feeling of love and compassion for self and others. While doing this, it also helps to create a positive mood, beneficent outlook and calm inner self. Referred to as "Metta" in the ancient Pali language, it is not intended to be used only for family and close friends but rather to extend to include others without any expectation of getting some reward or benefit in return.

This meditation is intended to bring loving kindness, compassion, concern, and care for one's own self and others. One must be comfortable and relaxed when practicing this method. While often practiced in a lying down posture, it can also be practiced while standing, walking, sitting and in any aspect of one's life.

Begin the process by breathing deeply, in and out. One should consider issues that crop up such as hatred, self-judgment and things you may want to improve. Starting with oneself, there is a repetition of phrases intended to be recited during the breathing process. While there are many variations on this theme, one generally asks:

- May I be free from mental suffering and distress.
- May I be happy.
- May I be free from inner and outer danger and harm.
- May I be free from physical pain and suffering.
- May I be strong and healthy.
- May I live in this world joyfully and peacefully.

From this starting point, there is a focus on others starting with those close to you in a positive way, perhaps a parent, grandparent, spouse or child. It could be a mentor or teacher of some sort. The phrases are repeated however this time as you focus on the person saying "May he/she be......". You finish your statements and now focus on someone you feel neither positive or negative about but in this case, instead of being non-judgmental, you focus on feeling positive about that person with love, kindness and compassion. You then turn to someone that you find difficult to deal with or have had hostile feelings about. Let the statements spread through your body as you muster positive energy and feelings and generate loving kindness to that person as well.

You can move to various categories of persons such as all humans, all men, all women, all animals if you choose but before you end, it is important to remain focused on positive thoughts and images concluding with "May all beings be happy, healthy, and free of suffering". You are free to make up your own phrases to repeat recognizing that the spirit is one of inclusiveness and kindness to all.

This method has been of proven value when skillfully used in incarcerated individuals who have a history of violent actions. Even though many of us have not committed crimes to this degree, we are all faced from time to time with feelings of rage, frustration, and anxiety. It is how we deal with these impulses that often determines the outcome.

Yoga

Yoga originated in India and refers to a mental and physical activity that can promote inner calm, increased flexibility, and improved muscle tone and control. Derived from the Sanskrit word "yuj", its literal meaning is "to control" or "to unite". Yoga is typically thought of as a series of exercises with various postures to be assumed; to those who know it more intimately, however, it can help shape your life and provide a structure for inner peace and happiness. There are several schools of yoga, each coming from a particular tradition and with its own series of practices. Most involve physical postures and methods of breath control. In certain circumstances, yoga has been linked to various religious practices and may be associated with "trance states" and spiritual exercises. Even the Zen Buddhist school of meditation has some of its roots in yogic practices and yoga is central to Tibetan Buddhism. That said, yoga is practiced throughout the world in a non-religious manner and as a way of finding inner calm and relaxation. While various books are available that describe the yoga postures and discuss breathing techniques, most find it best to learn from a skilled practitioner. This avoids the development of "bad technique" and also allows one to choose only those postures that are within one's physical limitations and reduce the risk of bodily harm.

Acupuncture

Acupuncture is a technique of inserting and manipulating very small gauge needles into specific points on the body along various "meridians" to relieve pain and exert various therapeutic results including fighting addiction. Some believe that it can also promote inner calm, though there are no randomized trials to support this claim. Developed first in ancient China, it is based on the belief that acupuncture points lie along meridians that carry "qi" or "vital energy". According to traditional Chinese medicine, one's health is a balance between "yin" and "yang"; acupuncture is thought to help regulate the flow of "qi" and blood in the body and thus provide a balance essential for proper health. Since disease states are thought to result when there is a loss of this balance, this branch of Chinese medicine believes that anything that helps provide harmony is beneficial including acupuncture, acu-pressure, heat treatment, and other therapeutic modalities.

The acupuncturist must decide what points to "treat" following a period of observation and questioning. Methods of inspection, auscultation, olfaction, inquiring, and palpation are used as part of the diagnostic process. Inspection focuses on the face and tongue. Particular details as to the size, shape, texture, and coating of the tongue are useful observations to the skilled practitioner. One's body odor and various sounds provide additional insights. Questions are asked regarding one's appetite, thirst and taste, bowel and bladder habits, pain, sleeping pattern, perspiration patterns, details regarding constitutional symptoms of fever and/or chills, history of vaginal discharge and menstrual cycle. Each treatment plan is individually tailored to the individual's unique characteristics and problems and is based on the practitioner's subjective and intuitive impressions. While usually considered as a possible treatment of physical ailments including pain, paresthesias, sprains, abdominal distention, arthritis, constipation, and other ailments, it is frequently used for treating addictions including smoking and drug. Increasingly, it has found a following in those with eating disorders, both anorexia and obesity, and in individuals suffering from sleep disorders, anxiety and panic attacks.

While there have been an increasing number of studies evaluating the potential benefits of acupuncture, little is known about the exact mechanism of action and not all studies are in agreement as to its benefit for specific problems.

Most studies to date have focused on physical ailments, particularly pain and treatment of addiction with little information to help evaluate acupuncture's potential role in treating anxiety and panic. Since muscle tension resulting from stress can lead to muscle spasm and pain and may be treated successfully with acupuncture, there may be a role for this ancient therapeutic modality in individuals unable to deal with the effects of stress in other ways and who suffer from its consequences.

Many believe that the insertion of these fine needles stimulate inner substances, perhaps our own endogenous opioids, the endorphins. Since studies have proven that even a placebo can induce an increase in the brain's release of endogenous opioids, there remain skeptics as to the value and physiological effect of the acupuncture itself. Studies using brain imaging suggest that the analgesia following acupuncture is associated with changes in the thalamus portion of the brain and various regions of the cerebral cortex. Studies have also demonstrated increases in nitric oxide levels in treated regions implying vasodilation and increased regional blood supply. Clearly additional studies are needed prior to making a more definitive conclusion as to the effectiveness of acupuncture and whether it is an acceptable way to treat a variety of conditions. There is general agreement, however, that acupuncture is safe when administered by well-trained practitioners who use sterile needles.

Tai Chi Chuan

Tai Chi Chuan comes from China and was originally considered to be a martial art. Tai Chi Chuan is increasingly used for promoting health and is gaining a great deal of popularity as both an individual and group activity. Tai Chi Chuan is derived from the Mandarin words "t'ai chi ch'uan" and means "supreme ultimate fist". The basis of this art is a variety of solo routines or "forms". These are based on body movement, changing posture, and balance. Focusing the mind on one's movements is thought to help bring a state of calm and improve one's ability to focus. It is thought to be useful for those suffering from anxiety and as a way of managing stress. It is also thought to improve balance and reduce the risk of falling among the elderly. The slow, repetitive nature of the movements are based on relaxation and not the tension and force of many other martial art forms such as karate. Loose and comfortable clothing and flat soled shoes are suggested to be worn during the sessions. The aspects of Tai Chi Chuan training, therefore, focus on relieving the physical effects of stress on the body and mind and allowing one to achieve calmness through the repetitive and meditative aspects of Tai Chi; Tai Chi's focus as a martial art is based on movements that allow one to move and thus yield to an attack rather than meet the force head on and strike using opposing force.

The solo form is a slow sequence of movements to be done with a straight spine; breathing is to be from the abdomen and a full range of movement is achieved with a focus on one's own center of gravity. This form of exercise develops flexibility as well as stability. Depending on the individual school of Tai Chi and the teacher, various speeds and shapes of movement from circular to square are used. Knees are also flexed at various angles to provide a low sitting and high sitting approach to the form being practiced. Another form is referred to as "pushing hands" and is based on balance and changes in posture. The philosophy of the martial art is that an incoming force should be met with "softness", allowing the person being hit to move with the force being exerted rather than meeting it with a firm resistance. If possible, the strike is to be redirected, thus reducing the impact that would otherwise occur. Through this activity, the goal is to exhaust the attacker and minimize one's own harm. The art is thought to "capture" the attacker's center of gravity. Advanced students learn to push and use open hand strikes, not punches. Kicks are directed to the legs and lower torso. Strikes to the eyes, heart, throat and groin may be given and in certain schools, weapons are used including the sword and wooden staff.

Modern Tai Chi is used throughout the world as a low stress form of exercise. It is particularly helpful for older persons who benefit from its focus on posture, emphasis on flexibility and rhythmic breathing as a way of inducing calm. While trends have been observed, scientific studies to date have failed to conclusively show improvement in flexibility, balance or cardiovascular fitness, as well as reduced rates of falling in persons using Tai Chi in their everyday life. Studies have also claimed its ability to reduce LDL cholesterol, norepinephrine and cortisol levels; these studies have been questioned in terms of their ability to determine if findings result from the Tai Chi itself or are consonant with that achieved with any form of exercise. Calorie expenditure from Tai Chi is similar to that one achieves with downhill skiing and thus is not considered to be a major factor in a weight loss program. One study reported that individuals who practiced Tai Chi who received a vaccine against Varicella zoster virus had higher and more significant levels of cell-mediated immunity to the virus as compared to a control population. No conclusion was able to be made regarding the clinical benefit from this laboratory finding though clearly additional research is needed.

Whether or not there is valid and significant physical benefit from practicing Tai Chi, its long tradition as a calming influence and as a way to possibly improve one's posture, flexibility, and stability, may be a nice addition to one's daily routine.

Find Your Own Prescription for Happiness and Calm

Whatever path you choose, remember that there will continue to be things that are out of your control. These factors will likely lead to stress and changes in your health if not dealt with in a favorable manner. You must find ways to accept these uncontrollable life situations and learn to deal with them in a more healthy manner. You must find your own prescription for health and happiness and the time to start is NOW!

Try one method and if it does not work, move on to another. Any of the stress reduction methods listed above may be used alone or in combination with others. A regular exercise regimen if done correctly is an excellent way to complement any of the stress reduction regimens though the goal is to have something that your body will learn to use without prompting and in any potential time of need. The key is to practice whatever you choose on a regular basis and incorporate it into your life.

18

Sleep: Necessary for Physical and Mental Well-Being

Sleep is a natural part of our daily lives and must not be taken for granted. We all lead busy lives and have many competing commitments such as family life, hobbies, and work just to name a few. Many persons wrongly believe that there is not enough time in the day to do everything they would like to accomplish and consciously decide to eliminate hours of much needed sleep, thinking that no harm will come of it. This is just not true and the consequences of too little sleep will become obvious if not in the short term, then over time, as proper sleep is essential if one is to achieve optimal health and a successful aging process.

There is great variability as to exactly how much sleep any individual requires. Most experts agree that eight to nine hours of sleep is the average amount that is necessary to provide the restoration of our bodily and cognitive functions and is necessary for maximal alertness, memory and problem solving ability and overall health. Less sleep has been associated with more accidents and an increased risk of developing certain illnesses.

That being said, there are individuals, particularly those over the age of 50, who claim to "function well" with as few as 4 or 5 hours of sleep per day. Of note, the average child aged 3–5 sleeps 11–13 hours a day; children 5–12, sleep on average 9–11 hours a day; adolescents sleep 9 to 10 hours a day; and adults sleep on average seven to eight hours a day. Several studies have reported that individuals who self-report sleeping between six and seven hours a day actually live the longest and elderly persons who sleep more than seven to eight hours a day reportedly have higher mortality rates. In fact, the correlation between lower hours of sleep and wellness in this older population only existed for those who woke up "naturally" and not with the help of some artificial means such as an alarm clock. Clearly, the reasons for the sleep pattern must be distinguished from the sleep itself and in no way should someone modify their own amount of sleep based on this data as sleep is a very individual process. Persons who have interrupted sleep, or medical conditions that promote more sleep may in themselves be responsible for the findings noted above.

We do know that lack of sleep increases one's risk of developing cardiovascular disease, weight gain, high blood pressure, and other illnesses. Wound healing has been shown in animal experiments to be affected by the amount of sleep and sleep deprivation has been shown to reduce one's metabolism and negatively affect the immune system.

Even if one gets an adequate amount of sleep, the quality of the sleep is also of paramount importance. Sleep is thought to be necessary for our process of cellular growth and rejuvenation. In fact, growth hormone, an anabolic or body building hormone, rises during sleep in our period of growth and development and is responsible for our achieving adult stature and development.

Even if one accepts that they need to obtain an adequate amount and quality of sleep, there are many obstacles for achieving this goal. Some of these include aches and pains, symptoms resulting from an illness such as a cough or sore throat, an itch, the need to wake-up to urinate, environmental disruptions, noise or movements from a sleep partner, anxiety or depression, effects of medication, and sleep apnea.

We have frequently noted the youth who sleeps through everything going on and well into the day on a Saturday or Sunday. We also have observed the older person who drifts off to sleep on a moment's notice, taking frequent naps throughout the day. The total amount of sleep one needs is additive; naps during the day will reduce the time one can sleep successfully at night, perhaps creating tension and stress on others.

With increasing age, there are changes in our normal patterns of sleep and likely there is a reduction in the total requirement for sleep, though there is a great deal of variability as to just how much is required in any given person. With age, sleep latency shortens and we also have less of the phase of sleep that is referred to as "deep sleep", the most restful sleep we have. The phase of sleep referred to as REM, or Rapid Eye Movement, is also reduced with increasing age. This is the time we dream. It is during this stage of sleep that many believe we resolve our daily anxieties, perhaps a contributing reason for the relatively high number of elderly persons with psychological problems.

An adequate amount of REM sleep is also important to our health and natural well-being. During our early infancy, REM sleep represents a majority of our brain wave patterns. The more immature the baby is born, the more REM sleep there is present. This is thought to help promote the activation of brain function. Studies in animals suggest that REM deprivation may lead to developmental disabilities during later life. It is thought that REM sleep is key to our memory and organization of knowledge later in life.

Physiology of Sleep

Sleep is divided into two phases, Rapid Eye Movement or REM sleep and Non-Rapid Eye Movement or NREM sleep. We cycle through these stages with the average cycle being between 90 and 110 minutes; there is a preponderance of Stages 3 and 4 sleep or "deep sleep" early in the sleep cycle and more REM sleep toward the end. Age, medications, illness, disruptions, and use of alcohol are frequent causes of an altered sleep cycle.

NREM accounts for approximately 75% of our total sleep time in normal adults. Non-REM sleep is classically divided into four stages. Stages 1 and 2 are considered to be the time we are in "light sleep"; Stages 3 and 4 are the time we enter a "deep sleep" phase and have what is described as "slow-wave sleep" waves on our EEG, a measure of the electrical activity generated by our brain. It is during these phases of sleep that we often have movement of our arms and legs and on rare occasions, episodes of sleepwalking. REM sleep is characterized by rapid eye movements and the relative absence of muscle tone. This is the time in our sleep cycle when we dream.

The four distinct stages to Non-REM sleep are characterized by the type of brain waves noted on the EEG. Stage N1 is delineated by the brain's switch from emitting alpha waves while awake (frequency of 8 to 13 Hz) to theta waves with a frequency of 4 to 7 Hz. It is at this time when we become "somnolent" or "drowsy". We may have sudden jerky movements to our limbs and also begin to loose our conscious awareness of our surroundings as we "drift off" to sleep.

Stage N2 is associated with brain waves between 12 and 16 Hz, known as "sleep spindles" and "K-complexes". This period represents 45 to 55% of our total time spent in sleep.

Stage N3 is associated with delta waves that are 0.5 to 4 Hz and comprise less than 50% of the brain waves noted during this phase of sleep. This phase is considered to be a "deep" or slow-wave sleep. During this time of our sleep cycle, we may sleepwalk, sleep-talk and have bed-wetting. Certain individuals also wake up in a "fright".

Stage N4 is characterized by a period of time in which delta-waves make up more than 50% of the brain wave patterns as we enter our deepest phase of sleep.

It is thought that both deep sleep and REM sleep are required for proper functioning. The more normal our sleep cycle is, the more rested we will feel upon awakening and the better we will be prepared for the day's activities. Clearly, disruptions in our sleep may lead not only to physical problems but emotional ones as well. Many a sleep partner has complained of their sleep being disrupted by their partner's snoring or movement. As sleep deprivation becomes a greater problem for both involved parties, tension can increase and with it significant emotional consequences. Sleepy sensations during the day may lead to shortened tempers, lack of an ability to concentrate or pay attention to what others are saying; clearly these and other side-effects are life-changing and place us at risk.

We fortunately can identify the cause of a sleep problem in many cases and treat the underlying condition. Sleep apnea is a frequent problem in obese individuals where the upper airway becomes obstructed, air stops its normal flow into the lungs, and sleep becomes erratic and interrupted with changes in the sleep cycle preventing a restful and rejuvenating sleep. Over time, this abnormal breathing pattern can also put adverse stress on the heart resulting in failure. Various oxygen delivery devices can be used to help keep airways open and thus reduce the periods of apnea that are the cause of the sleep disturbance. A trained professional can both assess the situation by doing a sleep study and prescribe appropriate treatment as necessary.

Medical problems such as pain or nocturnal urination may be disrupting one's ability to sleep normally. Here too, health professionals can assess the situation and offer treatment for the underlying condition. Emotional issues may also be presenting a problem to one's sleep and these should not be underestimated as a disruption of the sleep cycle will only compromise one's emotional state further. Speaking to a psychologist, psychiatrist, clergy member, psychiatric social worker, or member of the family or a friend may help one through the difficult situation that is affecting sleep; medications may also be necessary depending on how significant the problem is and its ease of resolution.

Sleeping medications are all too often thought of as a panacea. While they may help one fall asleep or keep one sleeping for a certain number of hours, most are addicting either physically or at least psychologically and many will interfere with the normal sleep-wake cycle or interrupt the normal stages of sleep with resultant consequences. Commonly, sleeping aids result in a loss of the ability to dream or result in more vivid dreams, at times even nightmares.

If you feel that you are not waking up "refreshed" and ready to approach the day with full vigor and enthusiasm, try to identify why this may be happening. Make sure you have proper "sleep hygiene", a comfortable bed, no disruptions, proper temperature in the room, comfortable sleep clothing, darkness, and a mental state of "calm and relaxation". You many need to refresh your memory of the Mind-Body relationship and develop your own method to wind-down for the night ahead and put anxieties and thoughts to rest. The same is true if you find yourself waking up early with anxiety and concern over events in your life. These must be dealt with successfully if you are to sleep normally. Some persons are overly disturbed by environmental noises and require a "white noise" to help them sleep. This may be in the form of sounds such as flowing water, waves, rain, birds, background "noise", or whatever else that individual finds best able to block out the noises that they find disturbing. Often a trial is necessary to find what works best for a given person.

If these methods do not work or you are unable to identify a physical or psychological reason explaining why you cannot attain an adequate amount of sleep, speak to your physician who may have additional insight and be able to offer you assistance. Help is available but you must seek it. While many persons try to dismiss their sleep problem as being a necessary compromise for the lifestyle they wish to lead or attempt to deal with the loss of proper sleep by using caffeinated products or medications to "stimulate" them to be awake, these are not the answer! An adequate amount of high quality sleep is necessary for optimal health and a successful aging process.

19

Exercise: An Essential Path to Successful Aging

Regular exercise has been shown to promote health throughout life and to help maintain muscle mass, body weight, mobility, reduce risks of falling, improve bone strength, increase bowel motility, optimize sexual function, and promote psychological well being. Unfortunately, many persons wait until middle or late life to begin jogging, bicycling, or even walking. While years of lost muscle tone and mass may not be as easy to rebuild, it is never too late to start a regular program of exercise. Physical activity alone will rarely lead to sustained weight loss or reduce one's high blood pressure and cholesterol level; nevertheless, it is an essential component of a healthy lifestyle and complements almost everything else that we do to remain healthy and happy. Too much exercise, however, is not a good thing and may lead to harm, muscle injury, fatigue, and burn out. Fortunately, we can achieve a great deal with moderate exercise, something within the reach of most persons. A regular and consistent program of moderate exercise can help improve our uptake of blood sugar into our body organs and tissues and reduce the risk of developing diabetes mellitus. It may also reduce the risk of heart disease and increase our endurance. Exercise, particularly that considered to be weight-bearing, helps keep minerals on our bones and helps us avoid developing osteopenia and osteoporosis. It also reduces our risk of falling and helps us develop better balance. It can also help us lose weight as muscle is a major determinant of our metabolic rate not to mention having a positive effect on our mental health, feelings of well-being, and confidence.

Exercise is an essential part of any diet as it not only burns up "additional calories" to help promote weight reduction, but also increases muscle mass. Muscle weighs more than fat but increases one's metabolic rate and promotes weight loss over time, especially the loss of unwanted fat. Most persons prefer the "look" of a muscular physique as well though depending on the type of exercise chosen, one can increase muscle tone and strength without "bulk" or achieve any combination of the two.

It is not uncommon for someone who is dieting and exercising to actually not lose weight to the same degree initially as someone of similar size and requirements who does not exercise; the person exercising may even gain some weight as they increase their metabolically active muscle mass. For this reason, monitoring weight loss too aggressively may be misleading. Exercise is the cornerstone of all weight reduction efforts and health promotion programs and must not be minimized!

Exercise can be tailored to meet your individual interests and abilities and can be advanced based on individual progress and goals. The nice thing about exercise is that there is no minimum level below which there is no benefit. Exercise has direct effects on our muscles and bones and also stimulates certain brain substances including beta-endorphin and growth hormone.

We are said to be "fit" when we able to perform our daily tasks in an efficient and active manner with sufficient energy left over to continue to enjoy leisure-time activities yet still have the reserve to respond to emergent situations. Fitness is a major foundation for being in good health and feeling "well". It involves proper function of the heart, lungs, muscles and even mind and interacts with our mental outlook and feeling of emotional well-being. It has no specific criteria that are universally accepted and varies from person to person as to when this state has been achieved. It is influenced by experience, genetics, diet, age, lifestyle, and physical routine and most importantly, it is something that each of us can control and improve.

The American Council on Exercise, America's non-profit organization that promotes fitness, has continuously supported the need to fight the growing trend of obesity in the United States. This effort has the support of the U.S. Department of Health and Human Services (HHS). A study conducted by the Centers for Disease Control and Prevention reported that deaths due to poor diet and physical inactivity rose by 33% over the past decade and will soon overtake tobacco as the leading cause of preventable death.

In the year 2000, there were 400,000 deaths in the U.S. or 17% of all deaths attributed to poor diet and physical inactivity. This is second to tobacco, but not by much with tobacco related deaths reported at 435,000 in the same year. What is most frightening is the rapid rise that has occurred in recent years. A public ad campaign designed by HHS is trying to increase awareness of the importance of exercise as a way of combating obesity and as part of a healthy lifestyle. While there is a particular focus on obesity in children, the message is clear — Americans need to lead more active, healthy lifestyles. Approximately 25% of Americans report doing little if any physical activity on a regular basis.

Most importantly, individuals should choose those activities they enjoy doing and that can be incorporated into their daily routine. Brisk walking is still the most common choice as it can most easily be incorporated into one's daily activities, has no start up expense, and has a low rate of injury associated with it. For those who have the motivation, however, an individualized exercise program can be easily designed to meet specific goals. In addition, certain individuals are better "suited" to specific exercises and thus these will have a greater chance of remaining a part of one's lifetime routine. There are several "types" of exercise that one should consider prior to embarking on a specific exercise program.

Exercise can also improve functional ability and reduce the chances of falling in older persons as well as maintain and enhance cognition across the life span. Studies suggest that aerobic training programs combined with resistance training have a greater positive effect on cognition than aerobic training alone.

There are certain key principles to exercising correctly. First of all, remember that physical activity does not have to be strenuous in order to have significant and measurable health benefits. Men and women of all ages can benefit from regular exercise no matter how brief. Even the process of performing household chores has been shown to have beneficial effects on bone mass when studied in a group of older women as compared to those who led more sedentary lives.

Why is exercise so important? It improves one's quality of life, extends lifespan and helps prevent heart disease, high blood pressure, obesity, osteoporosis, diabetes, and one's mental outlook. It improves mobility, flexibility, and reduces the chance of falling later in life. Older persons who have a regular exercise routine tend to remain independent for a longer period of their lives and enjoy a greater number of activities, have better sex lives, and report a greater feeling of "wellness".

A fitness program can be achieved in a number of ways but to be complete it should lead to improvement in cardiopulmonary function and reserve; increased muscle strength and endurance; a greater degree of flexibility; a desired change in body shape and composition; and lastly, a feeling of accomplishment and hopefully inner peace. Cardiopulmonary improvement results in a greater ability to deliver oxygen and other necessary nutrients to the various tissues in the body. It also allows us to better rid ourselves of toxic wastes and by-products of our metabolism.

Muscle strength can be measured and is our ability to exert a "force" against a specific resistance. Muscle endurance is the ability of a muscle or group of muscles to be able to contract or act against a resistance for a measurable period of time. Flexibility is the ability to move joints and muscles through a full range of motion and relates to balance and agility.

Aerobic Exercise as defined by the American College of Sports Medicine (ACSM) refers to any activity that uses large muscle groups, can be maintained continuously, and is rhythmic in nature. This form of exercise is excellent for burning excess calories and has major benefit to the heart and lungs. It also has psychological benefits with most noting a change in their mood within

15–20 minutes of starting. This effect likely results from certain neuroendocrine changes that accompany exercise. The body's endogenous opioid system (the endorphins), growth hormone, catecholamines (epinephrine and norepinephrine), and ACTH, the body's stimulus to our corticosteroid production, all rise with exercise to varying degrees. While this is likely a natural response and a survival advantage as part of our "fight or flight" response to apparent stress, it also may be responsible for "runner's high", a term often described as the "incredible rush" accompanying exercise. It is this "endorphin rise" that some feel "addicts" individuals to an exercise routine. While men have a greater endorphin rise in response to exercise as compared to pre-menopausal women, post-menopausal women have been described as having a similar response to men. Animal data suggests that estrogens may limit this response; no data regarding this physiological response is available in humans to date.

As mentioned above, it is important that whatever exercise routine you choose, that it is something you enjoy doing, becomes a part of your daily routine or at least is done 3 or 4 times each week, and is capable of elevating your heart rate to a pre-determined level and amount of time. Aerobic exercises include running, walking, stair climbing, jumping rope, swimming, bicycling, dance, cross-country skiing, skating, and others. Some of these activities can be done with the whole family such as hiking, skating, bicycling, and swimming. Dancing offers a wide variety of opportunities including tap, ballet, belly dancing, jazz, country-western, swing, polka, line, tango, and others. Boating can also provide a degree of aerobic exercise if done correctly. This is most easily accomplished by rowing, canoeing, or kayaking. Safety and individual preferences and abilities must always be paramount in one's choice of a physical activity.

As one adds greater resistance or "weight" to the exercise program, as is the usual case with weight training (free weights or weight training equipment) or "resistance bands", an aerobic exercise may be converted to an anaerobic or isometric exercise. This form of exercise has the potential to build muscle tone and bulk but also has a tendency if too much weight or resistance is used to increase what is referred to as "afterload", the force against which your heart must pump! By using lower weight and resistance, however, one can add benefit to an aerobic activity while still minimizing cardiovascular risk.

While participation in group sports may have an aerobic component, they more frequently have "burst" type activity with intermittent periods of rest and thus may not achieve the consistent elevation in heart rate necessary for maximal cardiovascular benefit despite the caloric expenditure and feeling of well-being that may accompany these activities. By setting one's goals early on, it will become easier to determine what form of exercise will be able to help you to achieve the results you want. For example, if you desire maximal cardiovascular benefit, you need to increase your heart rate to achieve a minimum of 70% of your maximal heart rate (220 minus your age) for at least 20 minutes three or more times each week with some believing that: maximal benefit is achieved only by exceeding 80% of maximal heart rate. Clearly any man over the age of 45 or woman over the age or 55 years, or anyone who has a history of heart disease, diabetes, or hypertension needs to discuss their goals and the activity they plan to initiate with their physician prior to embarking on any exercise program beyond what they have been doing on a regular basis. A cardiac assessment may be advised prior to embarking on this activity. Those who have had any male member of their family die of a heart attack or arrhythmia prior to age 55 or a female member of their family die from a cardiac problem prior to age 65 are also considered to be at higher "risk" and are advised to discuss the new activity with their physician prior to starting. Additional risk factors include use of cigarettes, high cholesterol levels, and a very sedentary lifestyle to date.

Even those who cannot increase their heart rate to the desired "target" level for whatever reason can still benefit from more modest levels of increase and should not give up exercising in desperation. In time, additional increases may be possible but no one should exceed their limits or go beyond what they have been advised by their physician or trainer or feel is "right" for them. Listen to what your body is telling you. Problems with breathing, any chest pain or discomfort, feeling of weakness or dizziness, or muscle cramp or pain deserve immediate attention and should not be expected as part of a normal exercise routine.

Motivation is key to any successful exercise routine. Every day, many individuals start a program only to quit soon thereafter citing a myriad of reasons including lack of time, expense, inconvenience, loss of interest, difficulty in doing the activity, low self-esteem, and other factors. In fact, almost half of those who start an exercise program quit within the first 6 months. Do not get discouraged if you do not see immediate results.

While we all lead increasingly complex and busy lives, it is necessary to prioritize and commit the time necessary to achieve one's exercise goals; this time should be scheduled and agreed upon with all concerned. The American College of Sports Medicine suggests that an exercise session should ideally last between 20 and 60 minutes and occur 3 to 5 times each week. Sufficient time needs to be planned for any additional time spent in preparation, such as changing clothing, showering, and any necessary travel. Some individuals like to exercise at the beginning of the day while others prefer to exercise in the evening either before or after dinner. It is essential that one has the "energy" for the exercise program; avoid exercising after any prolonged period without food as well as immediately after a large meal. What works for one person may not necessarily be satisfactory for another. Experiment as to what "works" best for you. Exercising within two hours of sleep has been shown to potentially disrupt one's ability to fall asleep and may not be a good time for some.

Those who complain that they do not have money to exercise have not explored enough options or are too hung-up on status. Money should NEVER be a reason NOT to exercise. Walking, jogging, dancing and running are excellent cardiovascular workouts that are free and other types of exercise such as bicycling, cross country skiing, jumping rope, among many other forms of activity have minimal cost. Those who desire to exercise individual muscle groups and also want to increase the tone and strength of specific muscles can also do so with minimal cost by using easily obtainable and inexpensive elastic bands or even isometric activities that require no equipment.

Many individuals find that they exercise best when doing so with a training partner or in a group environment. It is amazing how motivated someone can become when seeing others doing a similar activity with the same goals and yes, problems. Adherence is also improved when you know that another person is counting on you for support and encouragement. Elicit the help of your family and friends as well. Do not feel that you are "cheating" them of your time, as the benefits noted will clearly serve you all well for years to come with better health and outlook.

Where you choose to exercise will also help determine if your exercise routine will succeed. Explore your neighborhood, local parks, waterways and determine if the path you choose is a safe one. Choose low crime areas and avoid high trafficked streets. Those who live in areas of the country that have harsh summers or winters will need to consider alternate ways to exercise during these seasons.

If a gym and fitness club is your choice, ask for a trial workout, speak to current members, and ask for a formal tour to become acquainted with the facility, its equipment, rules and policies. Make sure that the club meets your individual needs and is easy to get to within a reasonable amount of time during the part of the day you plan on being there. Some individuals prefer to go to a uni-sex club while others prefer co-ed arrangements. Find out if the club caters to a particular age group; there are suitable changing and grooming facilities; there are sufficient parking facilities and enough equipment available during the hours you will exercise. Some may want the services of a personal trainer, racquetball facilities, or spa-like programs including massage, sauna, and personal care; others may want a swimming pool.

Call your Parks and Recreation Department, YMCA, or local school to find out if any programs or classes may exist that interest you such as jazzercise, dance, yoga, aerobics, cycling clubs, swimming, among others. See if a friend may be interested in joining you in exercising. Some find it helpful to keep an exercise journal as a way of motivation; keep a log of your progress, goals, and any problems you may encounter.

Choosing to exercise at home is always the easiest but you must make sure that you have the proper motivation and if necessary, equipment to achieve your goals. Home exercise equipment can be obtained and varies in complexity and price depending on your choice. As mentioned previously, "elastic bands" can provide sufficient resistance training to increase muscle tone and even some bulk to muscles if desired and may complement an aerobic training program that uses a treadmill or elliptical training apparatus. Elliptical training reduces the wear and tear on joints by allowing one to "run" and achieve cardiovascular benefit though without the "pounding" accompanying treadmill running. The legs move in a rhythmic fashion on the elliptical device and most machines can increase the resistance that one must move their legs through and pattern of movement to even mimic a stairmaster effect. Given the choice of a treadmill or ellipse machine, the latter is preferable in terms of long term safety for the knee and hip joints though cost is a considerable factor to consider as treadmills can be purchased at much lower cost depending on the model chosen.

How to Begin?

Most exercise authorities recommend beginning an exercise program by first defining your goals. What will work for one person may be a sure way to disaster for another. Many factors go into what type of exercise program one would benefit from most including personality, body habitus, and prior experiences. Exercise goals should be specific, realistic, and include measurable outcomes. If weight loss is to be one goal, determine just how many calories you hope to "burn" to augment your diet plan and then choose the exercise regimen to accomplish this goal. Is your goal to change your physique, loose that "pot belly" or become more sculpted? Exercises can be individually chosen to achieve each goal as well. If you have not been active, start at a modest level and increase your level of intensity slowly. Monitor your pulse, breaths, and how you "feel". Do not over-exert yourself; remember it is not necessary to exhaust yourself or to harm yourself in order to benefit. The expression "no pain, no gain" is just NOT true in this case.

While the improvement you have in endurance and fitness will vary somewhat with your initial level of fitness, it is always possible to improve one's performance and to show demonstrable progress. It is also NEVER TOO LATE to start exercising to have a benefit as long as you choose your program wisely and base it on your own limitations and goals.

Many individuals are confused by the term "weight bearing exercise" and insist on weight training programs that actually may do them more harm than benefit. This is particularly true when considering an exercise program to maximize mineral content on bone. Weight bearing exercise is essential to achieve maximal effects but remember, your own body has weight and merely raising your arms through a series of exercises, perhaps holding a light weight, can provide the benefit you seek. Swimming, while a great aerobic exercise and one that can help burn calories and increase cardiovascular fitness, is not a weight bearing exercise and thus does not benefit bone mineralization as much. Choose your desired exercise after carefully defining your goals.

I am reminded of a patient I saw: Mrs. S was a middle-aged woman who was 4 feet 10 inches tall and weighed less than 100 pounds. She had significant osteoporosis and required medication and weight bearing exercise to help re-build her skeleton. Her husband, a large built weight lifter, insisted that she go to a gym and do free weight exercises; they proudly delineated how much weight she could "jerk" and "bench press" as part of her "weight bearing exercise program". Clearly this additional strain on her already frail skeleton was not "what the doctor ordered" and I tried to emphasize that this type of exercise was not only unnecessary but also dangerous given her frail bone structure and the increased risk of a vertebral fracture that her training could precipitate. I found out later that the husband refused to let his wife return to see me for her osteoporosis believing that he was "right". More is not always better when choosing an exercise program and goals for the exercise training must be clearly established. Too much exercise may also result in muscle strain, tears, and joint and ligament problems without added benefit.

The American College of Sports Medicine and the U.S. Centers for Disease Control and Prevention recommend the following for those who wish to increase their physical activity as part of a normal routine:

"Accumulate 30 minutes or more of moderate-intensity physical activity over the course of most days of the week".

For those who cannot add at least 30 minutes of a planned exercise or recreational activity, it has been suggested that one try to incorporate more activity into your daily routine including walking stairs instead of taking the elevator; raking leaves; gardening; dancing; mall walking while shopping; carrying a grocery basket rather than pushing a cart as much as possible; park in the most distant parking space available and walk to your destination. Be creative! While these activities can provide measurable benefits to your health, there is much to be said for incorporating a more comprehensive exercise program into your daily routine. In addition, maximal cardiovascular benefits require a more sustained and intensive effort than is achieved by most of the above measures. The choice is yours to make!

Recent data suggests that walking 10,000 steps a day regardless of the speed or distance covered and as part of any activity provides significant health benefit and should be a goal for us all. By using a simple to use pedometer, one can easily keep track of steps taken and adjust activity to achieve this goal. For most people, these many steps will be a stretch, at least early on. With time, however, and changes in routine and lifestyle, it can be achieved and become second nature. This does not mean that walking a smaller number of steps has no benefit as any increase in activity has its own rewards and provides a new foundation upon which to build.

Depending on your chosen exercise, you will reap different benefits. Many use exercise as an adjunct to a diet plan. Anytime your body "burns" more calories than it consumes, you will be in a negative calorie balance and over time, you will lose weight. In the short term, the body will strive to maintain a balance, but weight loss will result if you are able to maintain this excess calorie expenditure. The following is an estimate of calories used doing various exercises:

Type of Exercise	Approximate Calories used in 30 minutes	
	Men (175 lbs)	Women (135 lbs)
Basketball	330	260
Bicycling at moderate speed (12–14 miles per hour):	330	260
Canoeing/Rowing	290	225
Circuit Training	330	260
Dancing (ballet, modern)	250	195
Frisbee	125	100
Gardening	210	160
Hiking	250	190
Household chores (mop floors, wash car)	188	145
Household chores (dusting, vacuuming)	100	80
Jogging	290	225
Kayaking	210	160
Mowing Lawn-hand mower	250	190
Running (6 miles per hour)	420	325
Skating	300	225
Skiing (cross country)	350	310
Soccer	300	225
Softball/Baseball	200	160
Swimming laps	335	260
Tennis	300	225
Walking (4 MPH)	170	130
Walking — leisure	150	115

Flexibility

While aerobic exercise may have many benefits including improved muscle strength and a greater degree of flexibility for our muscles, joints, tendons, and ligaments, it is not specifically designed with these goals in mind. Flexibility is best attained with the use of specially designed stretching exercises. Stretching improves flexibility allowing you to move your joints through their full range of motion. It can improve physical performance and help relieve muscle stiffness that increases one's chances of injury. In fact, most exercise specialists recommend starting every exercise routine with stretching as a way of reducing strain and tears. Stretching helps lengthen your muscles and tendons while also preparing them for more intense activity to follow.

Most people find that stretching exercises provide a time for contemplation and relaxation while also promoting improved range of motion and flexibility. Many use some form of stretching to reduce stress; emotional stress is frequently associated with muscle tension and an elevation in blood pressure. In fact, many individuals who are under a lot of stress will complain of a headache that has as its cause muscle spasms in the neck region that radiate to the head. A controlled exercise that contrasts periods of muscle strain and relaxation is also often taught as a method of relaxation. The individual is taught to tighten a specific muscle or group of muscles in response to a stressful stimulus and then to "let go" and note the "contrast" between the tension and state of relaxation.

In addition to starting every exercise routine with a brief period of stretching, some advocate including a series of stretching exercises at least three times every week. Each stretch is aimed at moving a muscle through its full range of movement until you feel resistance, but no pain. This position should be held for a period of time ranging from 10 seconds in the beginning to 30 seconds after practice. You should then relax and repeat this motion three to four times. While some trainers suggest holding a "stretch" for as long as one to two minutes, this method is controversial and not universally accepted.

Avoid stretching too rapidly, but rather allow a smooth and steady transition. Limit muscle groups being stretched to achieve maximal effect and breathe normally during each movement, breathing "in" through the nose slowly and "out" through the mouth as you count through each stretching exercise. Do not hold your breath during a stretch. While stretching is strongly recommended prior to exercising, many believe that stretching is also beneficial after exercising to prevent muscles from tightening up.

Avoid what is commonly referred to as "ballistic stretching" or bouncing, repetitive movements done in concert with stretching activity. This may actually do more harm than good as these motions tend to shorten muscles rather than lengthen them which is the goal. Too vigorous stretching or holding the stretch too long can also be harmful and should be avoided.

The following are several popular stretching exercises that utilize a variety of muscle groups and body regions:

- Butterfly Stretch
- Chest Stretch
- Neck Stretch
- Spinal Stretch
- Hamstring Stretch

- Calf Stretch
- Shoulder Stretch
- Quadriceps Stretch
- Forearm Stretch
- Triceps Stretch
- Back/Lumbar Stretch
- Inner Thigh Stretch
- Outer Thigh Stretch
- Hip Stretch

Isometric versus Isotonic Exercises

Isometric exercises allow a muscle to contract without significant movement. This is also known as "static tension". This is in contrast to isotonic exercises that allow a muscle to contract with movement against a natural resistance. While these terms may be confusing and "iso" is derived from a word that means "same", isotonic exercises allow a muscle to change length and undergo a natural movement and are most commonly "aerobic" in nature and better able to promote cardiovascular health. While both of these types of exercises can improve muscle tone and strength, in themselves, they are not designed specifically to maximize cardiovascular fitness or as a way of burning excess calories. They are best combined with an aerobic and flexibility training program for maximal benefit and success.

Isometric exercises have not received as much favor in recent years as they were in the past. An exercise can be both isotonic and isometric, however, depending on the amount of resistance that is used at any time. For example, training with lighter weights or other forms of resistance can be an isotonic form of exercise and if planned correctly can also provide an aerobic workout. As the weight or resistance becomes greater however, it may shift to and become an isometric exercise with muscle physiology now affected in a different way in response to the higher and more challenging weight.

Many sports teams have reported success using isometric exercise as a way to improve strength; time has shown us, however, that these exercises are not without risk and may not be the best choice for the majority of individuals embarking on an exercise routine and/or as part of a weight management program. Most problematic is the increase in what is referred to as "afterload" or the force against which the heart has to pump blood. This can be problematic particularly in older individuals or those with pre-existing heart disease or high blood pressure. Any lifting of an excessive weight that does not allow a full range of motion of muscle groups and results in a "strain" will have a similar effect to that noted with shoveling heavy snow. It is not by chance that many people die each year from heart attacks as a direct result of the isometric response to snow shoveling, made even more dangerous by the cold temperatures that constrict blood vessels.

Strength Training Exercises

Exercise may also be used to build body mass and strength. No, you do not need to have the shape of a bodybuilder similar to those pictured in Muscle Magazines and on TV to gain strength and a feeling of accomplishment and well-being. Men and women alike are increasingly aware of the potential benefits of exercise and are choosing to build strength as well as endurance. As we age, we all will have a loss of muscle mass. This is part of the normal aging process, but it does not have to affect physical functioning even during later years of life. By having a "reserve" of muscle mass, there is less chance of physical decline with age leading to immobility, falls, and loss of functional capacity. The additional muscle mass will also increase our ability to "burn" calories to a greater degree and help us maintain our weight, or depending on the circumstance, help promote weight loss.

Similar to starting on an aerobics program, individuals may need to discuss with their physician whether or not it is safe to embark on a strength training activity. Men over the age of 45, women over 55, and those with a family history of coronary artery disease before the age of 55 for men and 65 for women are considered at greater risk and should definitely seek "clearance". Individuals with any cardiovascular disease, chest pain, abnormal cholesterol, cardiac arrhythmias, hypertension, lung disease, diabetes, significant obesity, arthritis, recent surgery, or who are pregnant or within three months of delivery are also advised to first obtain medical approval.

The minimum amount of strength training suggested by the American College of Sports Medicine is eight to twelve repetitions of eight to ten exercises at a moderate intensity, two days a week. Clearly, the more days per week and repetitions one does and the greater the resistance that the muscles must work against, the more overall benefit of the program in terms of muscle development. Excess weight, length of work-out, or improper technique increase the chance of injury whether it is a torn or strained muscle, ligament or tendon, injury to the nervous system, or micro-fracture of the bone, proper technique is key to success.

In general, most experts recommend resting each muscle that you are training for one to two days before repeating the routine. This allows a "healing" process to occur in response to the muscle stimulus that has occurred and allows maximal benefit. Remember, the adage "no pain, no gain" is a myth. Some fatigue and discomfort may be felt, especially during the early stages of any strength training program, but if the discomfort is more than minimal or does not improve during the rest period, it is better to delay the next training session. Seek medical advice if the problem does not improve within the next few days. Better to be safe than sorry.

Guiding Principles to Strength Training

Muscles must be "stimulated" in order to maximize a gain in strength. This is referred to as "overload".

Active muscles must continue to work against a gradually increasing resistance to maintain the "overload" stimulus and hence the need to continue to add weight at periodic intervals as you become accustomed to the higher weight.

Strength training is dependent on the "maximal force" that a muscle must work against in order to induce muscle hypertrophy. This is in contrast to endurance training that uses "submaximal" resistance and is more dependent on the number of repetitions that the muscle must undergo.

Avoid lifting heavy weights without someone available to assist you in case you run into trouble. Many a weight lifter has incurred major injury by losing their balance and forcing muscles to react in abrupt and/or unnatural ways.

Always start each session with a lower weight than your maximal limit and build up until your maximum is reached, performing 8 to 10 repetitions at each weight level.

Start your work out with stretching exercises to promote flexibility, range of motion, and increased blood flow to the muscles.

Develop a routine that starts with large muscle groups and then moves to smaller ones.

After reaching maximal limits, reduce weight and allow a "cooling-down" period to occur by returning to lower weights and more repetitions.

Pay particular attention to your breathing. Avoid holding your breath as this may result in a "valsava" maneuver that can cause the heart to beat in an abnormal manner, reduce blood flow to the heart, and affect your blood pressure. Breathe in through the nose and out through the mouth, slowly, and rhythmically with each repetition. Allow your breath to "work" for you.

The American College of Sports Medicine in 1990 recommended that in order to achieve both cardiopulmonary and muscular fitness, some sort of strength training should be included in all fitness routines. They recommended a minimum of one "set" of 8–12 repetitions of eight to ten different exercises aimed at conditioning major muscle groups and repeating this at least 2 days a week in concert with endurance training. Depending on one's individual goals, the number of sets would increase and be done more days of the week while still allowing the muscles to rest in between work-outs. This is particularly important if one is using major resistance to build not only strength and endurance but also to build muscle mass. Know your goals ahead of time. Cardiovascular benefit can be achieved through a program of aerobic exercise that will also help promote weight loss even without exercises aimed at improving strength. The decision of what type of exercise regimen works best for you is clearly an individual one!

The American College of Sports Medicine has published weight training guidelines for specific training aimed to improve muscle strength and mass. While they recognize that more than one set may be beneficial, improvement in strength and muscle mass will not be in direct proportion to the number of sets completed. Most of the demonstrated benefit in terms of strength and muscle hypertrophy or attained mass will be achieved after the first set. In fact, they report only marginal improvement in strength when more sets of the same exercise are used for a specific muscle or muscle group. They suggest that those seeking maximal benefit incorporate two or more different exercises per muscle group and aim for between 2 and 5 sets. One study compared outcomes in individuals who used weight training on a regular basis to improve strength and muscle mass. After 13 weeks, there was no difference noted in strength or muscle mass between those who exercised using only one set as compared to those who did three sets of the same exercises.

The terms intensity, duration, and frequency are common to the world of weight training. For years, bodybuilders and sports authorities have noted that these aspects of weight training work in concert. For example, if one were to work out more times per week, the same effects could be achieved by increasing either the intensity or duration of the usual number of workouts.

Intensity refers to the amount of weight or resistance that a muscle must work against.

Duration is the number of exercises or sets that are performed.

Frequency is the number of times a week that one trains.

A specific level of intensity must be maintained in order to continue to keep the newly achieved strength and muscle mass that has resulted from the training program. While duration and frequency may vary and will influence endurance to a more significant degree than the actual weight used, a specific program must be instituted to achieve the goals that have been set.

Most individuals embark on a "progressive" intensity program that is based on a gradual increase in weight resistance over time. There is controversy as to whether it is the intensity or the duration and frequency that best determines the degree of caloric expenditure that will result from a weight training program. Weight training has an aerobic component, though not to the same degree for most individuals as other aerobic activities such as running, cycling, or swimming. It also has an anaerobic aspect. Anaerobic activity should not be underestimated in any weight management program as the stimulated muscles will continue to burn calories even after the exercise is over as the body builds muscle mass and muscles hypertrophy. This process takes energy and thus calories continue to be used.

For most individuals, a program that utilizes a balance between maximal intensity and duration is preferred. In general, after a "warm up set" using approximately 50% of the planned maximal weight, two sets of 8 to 12 repetitions each should be done. Some will vary the number of sets each time they exercise, though the key is to continue to progress in the workout while monitoring your goals. Some individuals with more limited time to exercise find that they benefit more by alternating their sessions between aerobic activity aimed at improving cardiovascular endurance with weight training that is aimed more directly at improving muscle strength and mass. The choice is yours — the options are limitless.

Individuals who discontinue an exercise routine will find that their increased level of endurance will be the first to go; any attained improvement in muscle strength will also decline though at a slower rate. The key is to keep active and to ensure a regular exercise routine that will allow you to achieve and maintain your lifelong goals.

Weight Training Exercises and Options

Many strength training exercises can be used and are based on using either free weights, elastic or metal bands, universal machines, or nautilus equipment. These latter methods allow one to lift against a resistance without the added risk of losing control as the weight is returned to its original position following the extension and return of the muscle group. For this reason, they have a tendency to cause less injury but do require knowledge regarding their proper use. Depending on the choice of equipment, they also can prove costly for someone attempting to do their full exercise routine at home. Most fitness clubs have an excellent variety of exercise equipment at your disposal and it would be worth your time and effort to learn about the many options available and what would help you meet your goals in the best and safest manner. Even individuals who want to exercise at home can purchase exercise equipment that may not be prohibitively expensive; it pays to seek advice and consult an expert prior to making any final choices.

Exercises that are basic to any strength training program include the following:

- Bench Press
- Bicep Curl
- Tricep Curl
- Squat
- Leg Curl
- Leg Extension
- Lat Pulldown
- Overhead Press
- Abdominal Crunch
- Dumbell Fly

These exercises were first developed using free weights though modern exercise equipment can mimic almost any exercise that has been designed to develop specific muscle groups. Depending on the amount of weight and resistance, these exercises can be used to increase endurance by providing a form of aerobic stimulus to the cardiovascular system as well as build strength and muscle mass for those choosing to do so.

Choosing the Right Exercise Program for You!

Every individual is created with unique abilities, personality style, and body habitus. Just as we all enjoy different types of music, flavors of ice cream, and colors, we also need to find an exercise routine that fits our "personality" as well as our abilities. We need to identify the exercise routine that will enable us to achieve our pre-determined goals. While there may be certain limitations depending on where one lives, available financial resources, and physical limitations, it is always possible to identify something that will allow you to meet your goals.

Many persons who seek advice prior to embarking on an exercise program are told to do three "sets" of each exercise, each being repeated 12–15 times. In most cases, a "circuit" or combination of individual exercises aimed at achieving a comprehensive workout is planned. The truth is that even one set of 12–15 repetitions will have benefit. Doing various exercises aimed at developing different muscle groups, each 12–15 times and increasing the resistance one must work against or weight being used, will help add lean muscle mass. It is amazing just how quickly you will feel the difference and "know" when it is time for additional resistance or weight to be added. Most importantly, the aerobic component of the work-out should be at least 20 minutes in duration, preferably 30 minutes, and designed to end with a light sweat or if you are able to monitor your pulse, a heart rate between 60–80% of your potential maximal heart rate (220 – age), depending on your beginning health status, prior exercise history, and medical clearance. Exercise should be a regular part of our life, with the goal of completing a full workout three to four times each week.

The combination of aerobic exercise, weight and/or resistance training, and eating a proper diet is the most effective way to achieve your desired weight and body shape. After we reach maturity, our bodies do change in percent fat and muscle and our metabolism slows. Exercise and eating correctly can help you realize your goals despite the passage of time.

Both aerobic and anaerobic exercises increase calorie expenditure during the activity as well as afterwards. Aerobic activity is the best way to increase cardiac output and blood flow and by this process, metabolism increases and thus calorie expenditure. Weight training increases calorie expenditure to a smaller degree during the actual event, however, there is a prolonged calorie expenditure following this activity that is part of the process of building muscle. Significant loss of body fat requires sufficient intensity, duration, and frequency of exercise.

One pound of muscle burns approximately 30 to 50 calories per day as compared to one pound of fat that burns only about three calories per day. The more you build muscle, the higher your metabolic rate and calories used both at baseline and in response to exercise. While resistance/weight training can increase muscle tone and strength when done at sub-maximal forces, progressive increases in resistance can actually build more muscle to a greater degree.

The added mass may not fit everyone's idea of what they want for a final body shape. While many women may prefer to not have that "bodybuilder's" physique, and fear that weight training may have unwanted effects on their body shape, this is not a necessary outcome and should not deter any woman from this form of exercise as long as they discuss their goals ahead of time and seek advice as to what is the best plan for them. The use of lighter weights with a greater number of repetitions will minimize any "bulking" effect while still building muscle tone and strength.

It is interesting to note that most men will not be able to build large body-builder type muscles despite a program that involves heavy weight training; certainly significantly fewer women need to have this concern. The classic bodybuilder spends significant time perfecting their techniques to build muscle mass, far beyond what is necessary as part of a healthy exercise routine. They have often also used anabolic steroids at some time in their training to help stimulate muscle growth. Some bodybuilders may also have a genetic pre-disposition to maximally benefit in terms of muscle growth. For the rest of us, a moderate and well planned resistance and/or weight training program can yield desired results.

Remember that muscle weighs more than fat so it is essential to not be overly preoccupied with the scale when starting on a combined diet and exercise program, especially if there is a strong component designed to build muscle. Unwanted weight will be lost in time and the tape measure will prove success!

Exercises that build muscle and tone also help accentuate the body's natural curves and shape while also improving one's feeling of well-being and mental outlook.

Individualizing Your Goals

Exercise Can Improve Cardiovascular Function and Physical Endurance

Many individuals exercise as a way to maximize their cardiovascular function. Again, anyone starting an exercise program should first speak with their physician if they are considered to be in a "high risk" group as discussed previously. The heart is a muscle similar to all others in the body. While it beats continuously, it can still benefit from a controlled exercise that will allow it to beat at 60 to 80% of what it can achieve when beating at its maximum. Over time, this increase in "efficiency" will allow the heart to pump a greater amount of blood through the body with less effort, thus improving physical endurance. If carried out successfully, climbing stairs, walking at a brisk pace and even jogging no longer has to be limited by a feeling of a racing heart or being short of breath. The improvement will be gradual but steady and soon you will notice the difference.

Exercise will also help improve endurance by improving your lung function. This is done by increasing the tidal volume, or amount of air that the lung is capable of moving minute to minute with each breath. Dead space in the lungs will diminish over time as you notice the improvement in your capabilities. Exercise will also improve your lipid profile as stated previously and thus indirectly also help to promote a healthier cardiovascular state.

20

The Role of Exercise in Weight Management

Many individuals start an exercise routine in the hope that the exercise will help "burn more calories" and thus help them to achieve the desired loss of weight. There must be a "deficit" in calories if one is to lose weight with one pound theoretically being equal to 3,500 calories. In other words, more calories must be used by the body than ingested if one is to achieve weight loss. Each person has their "own" metabolic profile and will utilize calories at different rates in response to changes in diet and activity. Individuals with more muscle mass tend to "burn" more calories for the same duration of exercise. This is particularly helpful to men who tend to have a greater amount of muscle mass as compared to women and thus a higher metabolic rate. Even here, one must not assume that moderate exercise alone will lead to significant weight loss for most individuals.

Basal Energy Expenditure refers to the energy you use to keep yourself alive. In other words, you will burn some calories even while sitting, sleeping and watching television. Your "basal" metabolic rate accounts for approximately 50 to 75% of the calories you "burn" every day and is necessary to do the essential activities of the body such as maintain an adequate body temperature, circulate blood, and eliminate toxic wastes. Your digestive processes alone account for approximately 10% of the calories you use each day as part of basal energy. Depending on the type of foods you eat, you may be able to modify the basal energy expenditure and influence your weight management program. Certain illnesses, such as hyperthyroidism, pheochromocytoma, infections, and cancer cause you to burn higher amounts of calories as part of one's basal state due to changes in metabolism and are frequently associated with significant weight loss despite maintaining one's usual consumption of food.

While there are many ways to measure an individual's "basal" metabolic rate (BMR), one way is by using the Harris-Benedict Equation given below. Men and women have different BMR's largely due to differences in muscle mass.

Men:

$66 + (13.7 \times$ weight in kilograms$) + (5 \times$ height in centimeters$)$
$- (6.8 \times$ age in years$)$

Women:

$655 + (9.6 \times$ weight in kilograms$) + (1.7 \times$ height in centimeters$)$
$- (4.7 \times$ age in years$)$

This formula requires a correction factor of between 1.2 and 2.5 depending on a variety of variables and thus proves to be quite inaccurate and clinically not very useful. When calculating one's caloric requirements, however, the BMR is only part of the equation. The degree and type of exercise one does, body composition, type of diet consumed, health status, and other less tangible factors, such as the individual's anxiety level, medication use, and genetic make-up all influence the "final" number of calories required merely to keep one's weight constant.

For this reason, and in recognition that without the use of a precise scientific measure of metabolic activity, any formula is at best 90% accurate; some have advocated using the following formula to determine a rough estimate of daily calorie needs:

Take one's weight in pounds and multiply by 13 for minimally active individuals and 15 if you consider yourself active; you would need to add additional calories if you are "very active". Some use the lower number for women and the higher number for men as a starting point. For the 150 pound man, therefore, this would yield approximately 2,250 calories and for the 150 pound woman, 2,000 calories. This is generally a good starting point and is usually within +/− 200 calories of one's calorie requirements.

This is not the number of calories one would need to lose or gain weight but rather the number that is usually needed to keep one's weight constant assuming a normally active lifestyle. The total number of calories would need to be increased if one were exercising regularly, muscular, or had any number of conditions that might alter calorie demands as mentioned previously. When choosing your calorie requirements in order to lose weight, you will need to reduce the number of calories you require as maintenance by at least 250 calories a day with some individuals needing to lower their daily calorie intake by

500 to as much as 750 calories depending on activity level, age, and metabolism. Reducing your calorie intake too much is not advised without medical supervision as it may lead to fatty infiltration of the liver and abnormal liver function tests, significant muscle wasting, and significant ketosis, acidosis, and electrolyte abnormalities.

The body strives to keep itself in a steady state balance and therefore adjusts its metabolism moment to moment, increasing or decreasing metabolic rates as changes occur over time. Catecholamines and thyroid hormone play key roles in this delicate balance. As we age, however, we are less able to "up" and "down" regulate our metabolism. We become more vulnerable in times of caloric deprivation, for example, tending to lose more weight than we would have earlier in life if our calorie intake dropped below its customary threshold for weight maintenance. We also are less able to "up" regulate our metabolism when confronted with more calories than we are accustomed to and thus tend to gain weight more easily as we age.

With increases or decreases in calorie intake beyond that which the body can adjust for, we lose or gain weight, establishing a new "set-point" or plateau. Checking one's weight too frequently is a sure sign of failure in any weight management program. We lose and gain weight as mentioned in a series of plateaus and thus it is important to be patient but steady on your path to success.

Many years ago, it was observed that older individuals had lower metabolic rates than those who were younger. It was felt that this age-related decline in energy expenditure was inevitable and inherent to the aging process itself. Since thyroid hormone is also a major determinant of metabolic activity, with hypothyroidism lowering and hyperthyroidism raising metabolic rates, researchers looked to the thyroid as the key to the aging process. In 1977, a study at the National Institute on Aging helped clarify this issue in healthy individuals of increasing age. Changes in metabolic rates that were observed across the lifespan were found to correlate with the decline in muscle mass that was noted to occur with increasing age. When corrections were made for these changes in muscle mass, there was little to no change in metabolic activity associated as a function of aging itself. Regardless of one's age, therefore, the more muscle mass we have, the greater our ability will be to utilize calories; this is just another benefit from having a regular exercise regimen.

Within reason, you can calculate the number of additional calories that will be able to be generated from a specific exercise routine over and beyond that of one's basal calorie consumption. The absolute number of calories used will depend on the intensity of the workout, how many times a week you are able to exercise, and the length of time of each session.

Even if the activity is the same, however, there are differences between individuals in the actual amount of calories that are consumed. As stated above, those with a greater amount of muscle mass will use more calories than those with less muscle mass even for the same activity. Men generally have more muscle mass than women and usually "burn" more calories even for the same type and amount of exercise. Genetic factors also play a role with some individuals better able to utilize consumed calories than others. This is a result of an individual's unique "metabolic rate", ability to alter the "turn-over" of endogenous catecholamines that adjust moment to moment metabolism, and one's ability to up and down regulate various aspects of thyroid hormone economy in response to meals and activity. This latter metabolic response involves changes in thyroid hormone metabolism itself that yields changes in circulating T3, or 3,5,3′-triiodothyronine, a hormone that is three to five times more metabolically active than its precursor, T4, or 3,5,3′,5′ tetra-iodothyronine. Studies in animals have also shown a reduced ability to regulate thyroid hormone in response to stress and dietary changes with increasing age.

In addition, we all have specific body shapes that are largely genetically predetermined. Some of us are tall and thin while others are shorter and more stocky. Many of us have a greater number of fat cells in certain regions of the body such as the thighs, buttocks or abdomen; these fat cells are formed early in life when our genetically pre-determined "pre-adipocytes" fill with fat. Once formed, these fat cells remain with us for life. We do have the ability to make them bigger or smaller depending on our caloric balance. Studies in the 1970's determined that "overweight babies" tended to result in "overweight adults". While this does not necessarily hold true for all, there is a definite tendency for those who have a greater number of fat cells earlier in life to have to "fight" to remain thin throughout their lives. Does this mean the journey to a thinner, healthier you is out of reach? Definitely not, but the journey may be more difficult and challenging and mandate a unique strategy to help ensure success. It may also be more difficult to lose fat in specific areas of the body that have more inherent fat cells without significant weight loss; this may be unrealistic for some and result in illness if taken to the extreme and losing undesired fat in all areas of the body is the ultimate goal.

Just as no two individuals are completely alike, not all fat cells are created equal making things even more complicated. Those individuals who tend to accumulate fat in the abdominal region tend to have more heart disease; those with fat deposits at the thighs and hips tend to have more insulin resistance and are more prone to develop diabetes mellitus and problems that result from high insulin levels and blood sugar. They also tend to have more hypertension.

While an individualized exercise program can be a very useful adjunct to a diet and promote a negative calorie balance helping us to lose unwanted weight, many individuals will still find that their body fat will remain in proportion to what it was prior to beginning the exercise program. Even emphasizing different exercises that favor a more localized muscle or group of muscles, the fat over that area will still remain and only be reduced in proportion to the total weight loss achieved. Be realistic in your expectations and don't be "too hard" on yourself; learn to accept who you are as an individual and individualize your own goals and expectations.

As one achieves a negative calorie balance, the body tries to conserve energy by adjusting its metabolism. As stated previously, in response to this caloric deficit, there is a decline in catecholamine "turn-over" and thyroid metabolism is altered to shift to a less metabolically active thyroid hormone. If a new metabolic balance cannot be reached through these natural defense processes, weight loss will occur. Unfortunately, the initial weight loss is due to a loss of muscle mass; fat stores are lost later as nature tries to conserve this higher calorie tissue for its last stand against starvation. If one were to continue in this negative balance even after our fat stores became depleted, key muscle such as from the heart and diaphragm would be lost and death would be eminent. The initial loss of muscle is primarily from what is referred to as proximal muscle, essential for walking and getting up and down from a seated position. It is for this reason that physical activity must be an essential component of any weight loss program; exercise helps maintain muscle mass and holds the key to maintaining strength, mobility, and well-being as we lose weight and achieve our goals.

CHAPTER

21

Body Composition and Body Shape Type

There are many ways to assess the components of your body. While this is not a necessary aspect of a weight management and wellness program, it does provide a baseline and basis for comparison. As we age, we do undergo a change in our body composition. This is not something to be feared, but rather a part of the natural process of aging. There is an approximate doubling of body fat between age 30 and 80; it does not necessarily mean that we are "fatter", though some people are, but we do have a change in our content of body fat. We also have a tendency to lose muscle mass. This does not mean that an older person cannot exercise and build their muscle mass even beyond what it was earlier in life, but for the same amount of exercise, there will likely be less of an ability to achieve the same result as was possible earlier in life. There is also a reduced amount of "fluid" in the body, what we refer to as intra-cellular and extra-cellular fluid. This mandates that the older person makes sure that they drink an appropriate amount of liquid to avoid becoming dehydrated. This is especially important when an individual exercises and is sweating from the heat or is dieting and consuming less hydrated foods.

Most assessment techniques for determining body composition focus on the amount of muscle and fat in the body. While there are sophisticated techniques that help quantitate fluid compartments as well, these are difficult for the average person to do and offer little in terms of guidance when embarking on a fitness program.

The "gold standard" for determining the content of fat in the body is underwater weighing. Although not easy to do and limited to experimental studies, this method is based on the principle of Archimedes. Anything submerged in water will displace an equivalent amount of water by weight. The larger the percentage of muscle and bone, or fat free weight, the more the displacement. Another way to think of this is that fat floats. The greater the fat content, the lighter the body is in the water and thus less displacement. This measurement depends on the ability of the person being tested to comply with the necessary procedure of exhaling air from the lungs as well as remain under water for a period of time. It also does require the necessary water tank and apparatus to determine the results.

Another method for determining body fat was developed by a Cornell University physiologist and is referred to as the Steinkemp method. It uses skinfold calipers at various sites to determine skinfold thickness. Calipers come in various levels of quality and include the Lange Skinfold Caliper, used most commonly in general settings, and the Harpenden Skinfold Caliper that has a greater degree of accuracy and is used by research scientists and exercise physiologists. These cost between $200 and $400.

Skinfold determinations were originally designed to measure fat content at over a dozen places around the body; more commonly, either 7 or 3 sites are measured for future comparison. In the 1980's, a study in the United Kingdom compared the various skinfold measurements used alone and in combination with underwater weighing and found that there was almost the same correlation to body fat if one chose to measure only the tricep skinfold as compared to more exhaustive measurements. This has become the standard that is currently used for those who still wish to estimate body fat and follow its progress using this simple and universally available method.

The seven sites that have been used by some in an attempt to be more inclusive include skinfold measurements from the abdomen, axilla, chest, subscapular and suprailiac regions, thigh, and triceps.

The series that uses only three sites includes measurements from the thigh, tricep, and suprailiac region.

If done correctly by someone skilled in obtaining these measurements, studies have demonstrated the accuracy to be within 3%. When this method was compared to underwater weighing, it had an approximate 90% correlation. There are tables available to compare measurements to other persons of similar height and weight; this said, these measurements are best used to compare the same individual over time if judged to be an accurate assessment of body fat in the first place.

This method for estimating body fat content while easy to do and relatively inexpensive, does not measure fat in the body other than that which is subcutaneous. It also may not accurately reflect the individual who has fat deposits limited to regions that are not being measured. For this reason, some thought does have to be given prior to using this method as the exclusive way to estimate fat. For example, someone with large fat deposits localized to the thighs and hips may not be accurately assessed if one were to measure only the tricep skinfold.

Many health clubs and individuals have bought scales that not only measure one's weight but also can determine percent body fat using bioelectrical impedence. The individual stands barefoot on a metal foot plate and an unde-tectable low voltage electric current is passed through one leg and allowed to return to the plate from the other leg. Since fat is a very poor conductor of elec-tricity, the electrical impulse will be inhibited in proportion the amount of fat in the body. The machine measures the resistance to the current and through this method determines the percent body fat. Depending on the type of machine that is used, accuracy varies between a reported 2 and 3%. In order to obtain as accurate a measurement as possible, it has been suggested that the individual avoid exercising for at least 12 hours prior to being tested, not to eat or drink at least for 4 hours preceding the test, and to urinate just prior to test-ing. Some report that alcohol use within 48 hours and diuretic use may also limit accuracy. Of particular note, this method tends to underestimate the fat content of very obese individuals and overestimate the fat content of very lean persons.

The DEXA machine, or dual photon densitometry, is widely available as a way to assess bone mass. Using two X-ray energies, it can also measure body fat and muscle. This requires specialized computer software that is not universally available other than for experimental use. This method takes only a few minutes and is considered to be extremely accurate. While it does expose the individual to radiation, the dose is extremely small and there are no pre-test requirements concerning diet, exercise, or medication use. The major limiting factor is cost as this is not an inexpensive test and while insurance companies may pay for an assessment of bone mass using DEXA for particular individuals, body composi-tion is not covered under any circumstance. For now, this method of determining body fat is largely limited to experimental use.

There are other less widely available ways that body composition can be assessed including the 4Pi Body Counter that measures minute amounts of nat-urally occurring radioactive potassium in the muscles as a surrogate for measuring muscle mass. This result is then evaluated using computerized mod-els with measurements of skinfold to estimate the amount of fat and isotope dilutions to measure intra- and extra-cellular fluid. Scientific studies have used the MRI, or magnetic resonance imaging technique, to obtain measurements of muscle, fat and bone and thus calculate body composition based on com-puterized data collection and analysis. This method, though expensive, provides measurements that are extremely precise.

Another less available and quite expensive device uses the displacement of air to measure body volume and estimate body components. Known as "Bod Pod", this device reportedly is accurate to within 3% and correlates greater than 90% with underwater weighing measurements. It does require a significant amount of skill to use this devise as changes in temperature, movement, or changes in breathing can affect the end-result.

Lastly, body composition can be assessed using a computerized system that uses a probe to emit a "near-infrared" light capable of passing through both muscle and fat. By measuring the amount of this light source that is reflected back into the probe and recording other data such as height, weight, age, among other factors, body fat can be estimated. Data suggest that this method is not as accurate as several of the others described and in fact has been reported to underestimate body fat by as much as 4% in obese individuals and overestimate body fat by a similar margin of error in those with low amounts of body fat.

Individualize Your Exercise/Fitness Program by Body Shape

Classifying individuals for one reason or another according to the shape of their body has been done for centuries and in fact was first described by the "father of medicine", Hippocrates. The German psychiatrist, Ernst Kretschmer advocated dividing individuals into several classifications including plump (pyknic); muscular (athletic); frail and linear (asthenic); and a combination of these classifications (dysplastic). In the 1940's, American psychologist William Sheldon received some degree of notoriety when he suggested that individual personalities were related to "somatotypes". He proposed a classification method to characterize individuals based on their specific type of body shape. This conclusion was based on his analysis of 46,000 photographs of naked men on whom he had specific body measurements. In his book, Atlas of Men: A Guide for Somatotyping the Adult Male at All Ages, he divides men into three categories based on their amount of fat and muscle. He concluded that the size of the individual was not important in his characterization but rather the "shape" of the individual. He characterized men along a continuum with three classic body types describing the extremes:

Endomorph: these individuals were characterized as being stocky, fat, and heavy with a "soft body" and "poorly developed" muscles. Other terms used to describe these individuals included "round", "barrel" or "pear" shaped. Their head was described as usually round and they tended to have "short" necks.

Mesomorph: these individuals were characterized as being "husky", muscular, and firm. Their shapes were described as "athletic" and being "rectangular" or "wineglass" in appearance. They looked "strong" and tended to have thick necks and cubical shaped heads.

Ectomorph: these individuals tended to be slim and tall with "slight" body shape, little upper body muscular development and poorly muscled arms and legs that tended to be slender and long. Their shape was characterized as being similar to a "rail" or "tube", without clear definition of particular body parts. Their faces were noted to be "thin".

Of course, individuals could be a "composite" of more than one body type and may even have certain characteristics of all three. Using a numerical classification scale from 1 to 7 for each of the three classic body shapes, individuals were scored 7-1-1 for an extreme endomorph, 1-1-7 for an extreme ecto-morph, and 1-7-1 for a classic mesomorph. A meso-ectomorph would score approximately 4-5-0 and a meso-endomorph closer to 6-4-5.

Each body type was characterized according to five measures of physical performance: strength, power, endurance, agility, and body support. The endomorph characteristically was noted to perform poorly and the mesomorph perform well in all of these areas. The ectomorph, on the other hand, was reported to have a high degree of endurance, agility, and body support but lack power and strength. It would seem that certain exercises and fitness activ-ities might be better suited to individuals based on their specific needs and capabilities.

What made Sheldon's method of classification so unique was his linking body type to personality. Endomorphs were described as being more sociable, fun loving, easygoing, and relaxed. They tended to have more emotional sta-bility and a feeling of security. They were described as loving food and having a tendency to strive for comfort. They also were thought to be more tolerant and forgiving.

Mesomorphs were noted to be more athletic, physically active, aggressive, and stronger. They had more energy and a sense of competition. They did not care as much about what others had to say about them and were very confident, at times even power seeking. They loved to take risks and were adventurous.

Ectomorphs, on the other hand were described as being quieter, introspec-tive, sensitive, and self-conscious. They liked privacy and tended to be less comfortable in group settings. They were also thought to be less willing to take risks and fearful of change.

As you can see, there is a great deal of overlap between body shapes and much room for interpretation. Whether the personality characteristics that have been described for each body shape are more fact or fiction remains a subject of controversy. It is clear, however, that not all individuals are created equal and that genetic differences and environmental exposures may influence more than just body habitus.

If body shape does influence personality, then it would make sense that the type of exercise that would benefit each of us and would be more acceptable to our unique abilities and interests would also be quite varied. Not all exercises suit everyone. Some individuals are better suited to activities that are group ori-ented while others best thrive by exercising in solitude. Exercises may foster endurance and muscle tone while minimizing muscular development and mass. Other exercises are best used to build muscle mass or "bulk".

Whether or not these same personality characteristics are associated with specific body shapes in women is less certain though clearly any individual seek-ing to exercise with this in mind can modify their exercise program based on their unique characteristics and goals.

Start by listing what is important to you in terms of your goals for your exercise regimen. Do you merely want to increase your cardiovascular endurance while maintaining your current weight? If so, you may need to increase your intake of certain foods to keep up with the increase in calorie demands. If your goal is to improve endurance while also losing unwanted pounds, a reduction in your calorie intake will likely be necessary. While some people are fortunate and the exercise in itself will help promote the desired weight loss, this is less likely to be true for those who are more than 10% over their desirable weight and a combination of exercise and reduced calorie intake will most likely be necessary to help you achieve your goals.

While it is improbable that a person who is extremely over-weight will become "skinny", achieving a weight that is acceptable and promotes health is within reach. Persons who wish to exercise to build "bulk" and be able to flash a muscular image, might be frustrated unless they are willing to devote a significant portion of their week to a weight training program. Even here, many individuals depending on their genetic make-up and underlying body composition, will be unable to add significant bulk to their muscles without unhealthy measures. Toning muscles and improving strength is a more realistic goal for most persons with the most benefit coming from achieving your desired weight and improving your cardiovascular endurance and health.

22

Taking the Next Step in Your Exercise Program to Attain a More Successful Aging Process

There is no ONE way to exercise and what you choose to do is entirely up to you. There will be benefit from almost any additional activity that you incorporate into your daily routine. Seek advice from a trained professional if you have any concerns or questions. Some prefer to start by exercising only 3 times a week and increasing over time to a daily routine. Remember that a minimum number of sessions and duration of aerobic exercise will be necessary for achieving cardiovascular benefit though any amount of exercise has some benefit and should not be discouraged. Remember that you may be better suited based on a variety of individual factors and preferences to one particular form of exercise regimen. Do not let opinions of others sway you from choosing the "right" program for YOU!

Some individuals believe that they will never be able to find time out of their busy schedules for a formal daily exercise and are happy if they are able to carve out time only a few times each week or use daily opportunities to increase energy expenditure such as walking up the stairs instead of using an elevator, among other easy to do adjustments to one's routine. Some people prefer to exercise with others around and find this "group dynamic" to be a stimulus to their routine. Others prefer to exercise in the solitude of their home, perhaps due to time constraints or a personal wish to remain private. Still others like to train with a partner, seeking mutual encouragement and assistance. There is no "right" or "wrong" way to remain physically active as long as one accomplishes one's goals and does not exceed one's own limitations. Just as we all have our own body-type and personality, we also have our own likes, dislikes, and abilities. The better you can define YOUR limits and establish a routine that will work for YOU, the better chance you will have for success and long term benefit.

Set goals for yourself and adhere to your chosen regimen; as long as you do this, you are on the right track. Some find it helpful to enter into a written contract, a commitment to complete a course of exercise. While only you will know if you do not achieve your expected goals, the commitment may be a useful way to help ensure compliance and keep you "on track". Make sure that your goals are internalized and that you repeat them as often as necessary to motivate yourself and keep you focused. Do not be concerned by what others have set as their goals — each person is unique and must have their own set of objectives to aim for.

Do not be afraid to set more modest, yet attainable goals to start with. You can always build on these initial goals as you progress toward your eventual endpoint. Do not be complacent, however, as what is gained can just as easily be lost by failing to remain on a maintenance program, discontinuing your routine, or skipping various regimens or stopping the routine completely for days at a time. Whenever you think of skipping a workout or some part of it, remember to focus on your eventual goals as well as look back at the workouts to date and how accomplished you felt when you last performed the task. This "image" can be a useful tool to motivate you in difficult times.

Always seek new and alternate ways to meet your exercise goals. By changing your routine, it becomes less of a chore and more of a challenge. Try a different form of exercise as long as the workout time and intensity is maintained. Experiment with challenging different muscle groups or using different rhythms, breathing techniques, or number of repetitions. If you prefer, use "number of steps" per day based on a pedometer measurement as a guide for your exercise goals. You are in control!

Keep a diary of your exercise, listing the date, time and duration of exercise routine, type of exercises you have done, number of repetitions and sets. You would be wise to record your pulse at the start of the exercise session and periodically during the workout. Record the pulse at the end of your session and then one and three minutes after its completion while you are resting. The more "fit" you become, the faster your heart rate will return to its pre-exercise baseline after the exercise session has ended.

Try to use exercise as a way to control everyday stress and in this way, use exercise as a way to improve both your mental and physical health. This technique is discussed separately in the chapter on Mind/Body. Just as when we eat, be Mindful throughout the exercise routine, paying attention to every moment and movement with full concentration and maintain a complete awareness of what is happening around you at all times. This method will help motivate you through your routine and will also help you to reduce your chances of injury and burn-out. The rhythmic breathing of an exercise routine can be thought of as a "relaxation technique" in a similar way one breathes to focus one's attention on the present moment during a session of Mindfulness Meditation. While exercise can be invigorating and strenuous, it can also be calming for both the body and mind!

23

You Are What You Eat!

Obesity Reaches Epidemic Proportions!

Perhaps one of the biggest challenges to the health status of our nation is the epidemic of obesity that has developed over the past few decades. True, we live in a more sedentary society, but that is not the only answer. More people than ever before are eating out and subsisting on pre-prepared foods. Portion size has grown dramatically in recent years and diets now consist of more refined sugars, fats, and most importantly calories. Obesity contributes to our nation's health care bill by increasing one's risk of developing hypertension, arthritis, heart disease, diabetes, and other health risks. Clearly, something must be done and the time is now! Obesity is a disease that can be prevented and treated at any stage.

What is a normal weight and how can we achieve desired goals? The Metropolitan Life Insurance Company has for years produced a weight table that provides desired weight ranges for individuals of varying height. While former tables took "body frame" into consideration, newer tables only consider height and age, recognizing that individuals that start out life thin and gain weight over their life-spans actually are better prepared during old age to fight infection and illness and actually live longer. The desired weight increase over one's lifetime that appears to be protective is in the 10%–20% range; higher weight gains are associated with reduced lifespan. Individuals who are more than 10%–20% below their appropriate weight for age may also be at higher risk of dying earlier. This has been described as a "U" Shaped Curve.

It should also be noted that not all weight is equal. Muscle weighs more than fat and one's fluid status also contributes to one's weight on a scale. How to achieve one's individual goal for weight is a very individual process and depends on genetic make-up, body composition, amount of physical activity, co-existing illness, and diet.

Not all bodies handle calories equally as well and not all food contains the same calories even for the same apparent quantity. In addition, the body utilizes calories differently depending on whether they are derived from fat, carbohydrate, or protein. Whereas 99% of consumed fat is utilized by the body and 98% of carbohydrate, only 78% of protein is able to be utilized due to the higher energy necessary to "break down" the protein bonds that form the food source. Even the way you consume the calories has an impact on your overall weight management. The body continually strives to maintain its weight at a constant level. Through a complicated process that depends largely on our "fight-flight" hormones, epinephrine and norepinephrine, and thyroid hormone, we are able to increase or decrease, depending on the circumstance, our "turn-over" of energy. This mechanism allows us to over-eat for a brief period and not gain weight. Similarly, we can miss a meal without losing weight. If this pattern continues, however, we establish a new "set-point" and our weight will change. This pattern was first observed over 100 years ago and was referred to as "luxusconsumption" or the "luxury of eating". We all have had experiences of eating that 3,500 calorie sundae with hot fudge, nuts, and whipped cream, fearing the worst when we next went on the scale. What a surprise to see the next day that our weight was still the same and we were none the worse for this brief, but pleasurable indulgence. Our fate would have been very different if the sundae became a regular component of our diet.

Similarly, we have all had to skip a meal due to some meeting or event and yes, our weight did not change either. Our bodies are amazingly adept at being able to maintain a constant weight despite acute changes in our diet and caloric intake.

This may not hold equally well for all individuals. It has been shown that older experimental animals are less able to "up and down regulate" their metabolism in response to over or under eating, respectively. It may not be a coincidence that older persons suffer more weight fluctuations in response to acute changes in diet than younger persons in similar situations.

Believe it or not, scientific evidence even tells us that there is a difference between individuals who "nibble" and those who "gorge" even if they consume the same amount of food during the day. The "nibbler" is constantly sending a message to the brain and regulatory hormones in the body that a steady metabolism is necessary; the "gorger", on the other hand, sends the message early in the day that there is some unnatural crisis and that the body is in a state of fasting or impending caloric deficit. This mechanism down regulates the energy burning components in our body in an attempt to conserve energy; when the food is actually consumed, it will be metabolized less efficiently. Over time, the "gorger" will have a greater caloric burden to deal with and has a higher tendency to become overweight or in the case of dieting, a harder time losing weight despite consuming the same amount of total daily calories as the "nibbler".

We are what we eat! But equally as important, we are a product of our genetic make-up. We are born with a certain amount of pre-adipocytes, each with the potential early in life to fill with fat and become full fledged fat cells. Once formed, these fat cells can get bigger or smaller, but they never disappear! With this in mind it is easy to understand just why "fat babies make fat adults". The early years are critical in shaping our lifelong body habitus and future health status. Foods we eat or fail to eat may have other consequences as well. Insufficient calcium intake early in life will reduce the potential bone mass we carry into adulthood. Genetics is also a major determinant of just how much bone mass we have at our peak with lower amounts noted in women of Northern European and Asian descent. It is this bone mineral content that helps determine, along with several other factors, whether our bones will continue to remain strong and fracture resistant later in life or predispose us to a greater risk of osteoporosis and fractures as we age. Men tend to have more mineral in their bones and thus are protected from osteoporosis under most circumstances; that said, a lifetime of low calcium intake, alcoholism, hypogonadism, use of certain medications such as steroids, among many other factors may also pre-dispose the older man to developing weaker bones.

Genetics also plays a role in exactly where we deposit fat in our bodies. We have all seen men and women who have large fat deposits in their abdomen despite relatively thin legs, buttocks, and thighs. On the other hand, many have a tendency to deposit fat on their thighs and buttock areas yet are thin at the waist. These individuals are metabolically as well as genetically different. The person who tends to develop central obesity (referred to as an "apple") has a higher pre-disposition to cardiovascular disease as compared to the person who tends to develop buttock and thigh obesity (referred to as a "pear"); this latter body habitus is more commonly associated with insulin resistance and diabetes mellitus. While we are not completely sure why central obesity has a greater association with cardiovascular illness, experts believe that fat cells deep in the abdomen secrete substances that are different from what is secreted by subcutaneous fat. Since this central fat drains directly into the liver, it is also thought to have a greater effect on cholesterol production. Abdominal obesity also may change the hemodynamics of our cardiovascular system by increasing the afterload, or force that the heart must pump against.

Women have a higher tendency to become "pears" whereas men are more commonly "apples" though this is not absolute. Scientific studies have demonstrated differences in the metabolic properties of the fat depending on whether it is distributed in the abdominal region or thigh/buttock area.

There are many health problems that have been linked to obesity. Some of these are listed below.

Obesity Associated Health Problems

- Type 2 Diabetes Mellitus
- Hypertension
- Hyperlipidemia

- Cardiovascular Disease
- Stroke
- Cancer (men: liver, pancreas, stomach, esophagus, rectum, gall bladder, multiple myeloma; women: uterus, kidney, cervix, pancreas, breast, liver, ovary, colon, rectum, gall bladder)
- Gastrointestinal disease (GERD, gastritis, gall stones, non-alcoholic steato-hepatitis)
- Kidney disease (kidney stones, chronic renal insufficiency)
- Infertility (polycystic ovarian syndrome)
- Endocrine Disorders (menstrual abnormalities, insulin resistance, diabetes mellitus, altered cortisol and estrogen metabolism)
- Osteoarthritis
- Sleep Apnea
- Pulmonary embolism
- Depression.

While behavioral and genetic factors are key to the development of obesity during one's life, social pressures, customs, and acquired habits also frequently contribute. Certain medications also promote hunger and may lead to weight gain.

Common Medications Associated with Weight Gain

- Thioridazine
- Resperidone
- Clozapine
- Amitryptyline
- Imipramine
- Paroxetine
- Valproate
- Carbamazepine
- Gabapentin
- Insulin
- Sulfonylureas
- Thiazolidinediones
- Cyproheptadine
- Propanolol
- Terazosin
- Contraceptives
- Progestins
- Glucocorticoids.

Regulation of Appetite

We are now aware that our desire to eat is largely regulated by substances in the body. These are not only produced in the brain, but also the stomach and pancreas. Years ago, I described a relationship between the endorphins, a component of our endogenous opioid system produced in the hypothalamus where it is thought the "feeding center" lies, and feeding behavior. More recently studies have identified other substances that also appear to play a role in regulating our eating behavior. One example is ghrelin. Synthesized as a pre-prohormone, ghrelin is broken down by enzymes to form a 28 amino acid peptide. Synthesis of ghrelin occurs in the epithelial lining cells of the fundus of the stomach with smaller amounts being produced in the kidney, pituitary, hypothalamus, and even placenta. Ghrelin in the hypothalamus is thought to play a major role in regulating our appetite as well as stimulating the production of growth hormone, an anabolic or energy producing hormone. Cells within the anterior portion of the pituitary gland have receptors for ghrelin and when stimulated there is a secretion of growth hormone. Receptors for ghrelin have also been found in the heart and fat tissues.

Ghrelin appears to have two main functions. It stimulates growth hormone secretion in concert with the action of growth hormone releasing hormone and somatostatin. It also plays a role in regulating energy balance by increasing our feeling of hunger; this is thought to occur through its action on the feeding center in the hypothalamus. Ghrelin concentrations increase during periods of fasting; exogenous administration of ghrelin leads to a sensation of hunger. Ghrelin has also been shown to stimulate gastric emptying and increase cardiac output. Ghrelin directly regulates the processing of nutrients by adipose cells thus helping them to store energy. This is done by alteration in the expression of genes that code for adipocyte enzymes involved in nutrient metabolism. Of note, although ghrelin has its own effect on fat metabolism and is lipogenic, promoting fat storage, it also stimulates growth hormone secretion from the pituitary gland with direct lipolytic action that promotes fat breakdown. Ghrelin also has been shown to activate cholinergic-dopaminergic cells in the brain that are also thought to play a role in the complex regulation of our appetite.

While ghrelin remains a topic of great interest experimentally, we do know that animals that have been treated in a way to reduce their ghrelin lose weight and fat despite eating a similar amount of food as animals that were not treated in this way. This has led some to propose that a vaccine against obesity may be possible sometime in the future. It should be noted that this is quite complex and we do not have all of the answers presently. For example, ghrelin concentrations in the blood are reportedly reduced in obese humans as compared to levels found in thin individuals. One exception, however, are patients with Prader-Willi Syndrome who have been described as having uncontrollable and voracious appetites and exceptionally high levels of ghrelin. Patients with anorexia nervosa, a disorder associated with pathological thinness and poor food intake, paradoxically have higher than normal plasma ghrelin levels; these levels decrease with weight gain.

Another substance of great interest is PYY-336, a hormone that makes one feel full. This is thought to function as an anti-ghrelin agent. As ghrelin reaches the brain and we become hungry, it is thought that PYY rises and leads to a decrease in appetite. It is this balance that is thought to be key in our weight control though there are many other reasons for eating, particularly one's state of mind and psychological profile. Of interest, lack of sleep has been associated with an elevation in ghrelin production, perhaps leading to increased appetite and greater food intake.

Leptin is another hormone that is thought to play a key role in the regulation of our energy intake and expenditure. It is produced by the fat cells themselves and was first identified in 1994 in a group of obese mice that had increased eating behavior due to a genetic factor. Leptin is coded for on chromosome 7 in humans and interacts with receptors in the hypothalamus, the portion of the brain thought to contain the appetite center. Leptin apparently is another signal to the brain that the body has had a sufficient quantity of food, a process known as satiety. If there is a disorder of the leptin process, there may be a dysregulation of our appetite and severe obesity may result though this is still the focus of research. Circulating levels of leptin are thought to provide the brain with information as to our energy stores and thus help determine our appetite level. Leptin, working along with insulin, appears to also play a role in our fat regulation and circulates in quantities in proportion to our amount of body fat. Why then is it thought that obese individuals have high levels of leptin, a substance in the body that normally sends the signal of fullness and a message to stop eating?

Although leptin helps regulate our appetite and plays a role in giving us a message that we are "full", in the case of obese individuals with high levels of leptin, the underlying problem is a "resistance" to leptin's action and thus the body's attempt to over-ride this process by having a relatively high level of leptin circulating in the body.

Individuals who are fasting or on a very low calorie diet have been reported to have lower levels of circulating leptin.

It appears that our eating behavior is quite complex and under the influence not only of environmental, social, and psychological factors but also a variety of hormones and peptides with often confusing and possibly conflicting messages. Additional research is clearly needed in this area prior to our being able to use the knowledge to our advantage to help modify eating behavior and energy balance.

CHAPTER

24

Choosing a Diet:
What Will Work?

What exactly is the "best" diet we can consume to remain healthy throughout our lives, insure that we remain fit and reach our weight goals, and live as long as our genetic make-up will allow? The simple truth is that there is no ONE answer and many options should be considered as the "right" diet for you. I must admit that I believe that a Mediterranean Diet that emphasizes ample amounts of fruit, vegetables, and whole grains and minimizes the intake of red meat and fat has stood the test of time as one of the best options one can choose to maximize health throughout life. Studies support its benefit on reducing the risk of cardiovascular disease, certain cancers, hypertension, and inflammatory processes. Even here, however, if one is not careful, excess calorie intake can lead to the accumulation of fat stores, insulin resistance, and health concerns.

Remember, as we age, our metabolism is not the same as it was during our youth and an adjustment in calorie intake and increased exercise may be necessary merely to keep our weight constant. Both of these will help to increase your ability to utilize calories as well as to build muscle mass, a major determinant of how well each of us can metabolize the calories we eat.

Keeping track of our weight, our ability to remain active, and our food intake will become more necessary as we cross over that threshold from our period of growth and development, to maturity and eventually, senescence. Unfortunately, many persons find themselves in a situation where they have gained considerable weight and now must take more dramatic steps to lose unwanted weight prior to going on a maintenance diet program. But beware! You will need to find a path that will provide you with a lifetime of good health and not just focus on short-term goals.

171

The literature is filled with many "quick-fix" diets offering solutions to our dietary problems. While many work for the short term, the true marker of success is a diet's ability to work in the long term and to promote health, not side-effects, accelerated aging, or disease. Any "successful diet" must not only help you to lose weight but maintain your desired weight for the long term while allowing you to maintain a healthy state and remain maximally functional throughout your life.

In some ways, we ARE what we eat — or fail to eat. The effects of over and under nutrition, however, may not be immediately noticeable. They may build up over time and affect the way we feel and/or function just when we need it the most — in our mature years. The reserve capacity we depend on during old age needs to be maintained and cherished if we are to live long, happy and healthy lives.

There have been many "flash in the pan" diet fads that have taken the country by storm. Some still enjoy popularity and each has a special "appeal" to the individual who has decided to "lose unwanted weight". Many persons, however, go from diet to diet, becoming disillusioned after the first few days or weeks; others find themselves gaining back the weight they lost initially on a specific diet as it reached the "maintenance phase" and decided to choose another, perhaps more appealing diet in the hope that this one would be "it". Individuals who find themselves on this unfortunate cycle, are more prone to have significantly reduced muscle mass and bone density and more quickly gain weight upon changing their diet.

Diets that focus on the "psychology" of eating recognize that many individuals just cannot resist that "extra" piece of bread or decide what is the "right" sized portion of food for them at any given time. With this as the over-arching goal, several diets offer pre-packaged foods/meals that help eliminate the guess work of how many calories are contained in any given food, how much to eat, and to simplify the choice of options. Diets that offer a liquid or a repetitive and fixed meal also play on this psychology as well as provide a reduced caloric intake. Many will include daily requirements of protein, fat, carbohydrate, vitamins and minerals while some may lack a specific nutrient. There is some truth that these pre-determined diets may serve for some people as a quick "jump start"; switching to a more balanced diet that can be maintained will be necessary for longer term success and health. Most individuals will not benefit with this as their only plan as it does not allow someone to lead a more normal life and the cost to purchase special foods that are required is often beyond the reach of the average individual. It is important to aim for a lifetime of proper and healthy nutrition; finding a diet that helps to incorporate healthful measures daily should be everyone's goal.

The average American has a major problem when it comes to choosing the "size" of their portions. In fact, over the past decade we have been conditioned to eat more and more — a product of the "fast food" revolution. The 1/4 pounder soon became the half-pounder, and then it was combined with bacon and/or cheese. We all know how hard it is to pass on that "large portion of fries" that is being offered for the same price as the usual small portion — a bargain or another "nail on the coffin"? 100 grams of one cereal may not provide the same quantity in a bowl as another cereal and who has the patience to weigh their food consistently. Purchasing a food scale may be an excellent investment to take the guess-work out of your cooking and as a way to help one plan a meal — clearly this will not appeal to everyone and is limited by practical considerations. Fortunately, once you have "weighed" a few portions of various food products, the desired size of each will become second nature. In general, a "portion" of meat, fish, or poultry should be the size of your closed fist; this approximates 3–4 ounces under most circumstances though it may vary from person to person.

Diets may restrict the amount of protein, carbohydrate, or fat; however, in order to lose weight, the mathematics is simple and fool proof:

> ### Caloric expenditure must exceed caloric intake.

Caloric expenditure can be increased by a regular program of exercise as long as the "difference" between calorie intake and expenditure is appropriate for the weight loss one desires. This has the added benefit, if structured correctly, of adding muscle mass. Since greater muscle mass increases basal energy expenditure, or basal metabolic rate, not only does one look better and have improved endurance and agility, but one's diet is further enhanced and more calories are "burned" for the same amount of activity. We have previously outlined what food and dietary components are necessary for maximal health benefit and what is best avoided; the choice is yours to make as you determine what you will be eating each day.

Eating less calories is not the only choice one must make, however, as not all sources of calories are created equal. Should one emphasize protein, fat, carbohydrate or some combination of these? This is where the diet game becomes even more problematic and almost religious in nature with "believers" and "non-believers".

My own personal belief is that men and women were meant to eat a diet that contained a variety of foods of different textures and constituents. Just look at our teeth — we are blessed with teeth that allow us to "tear", "chew" and "shred", unlike the majority of the animal kingdom. Most of us are equally adept at digesting and absorbing dairy products as we are fruits, vegetables and meats. It is by eating a variety of foods that we obtain our required mix of nutrients including vitamins, minerals, proteins and yes, even fats. That said, it is possible to eat too much of a given food source just as it is not good to eat too many calories, and not all foods are created equal as was noted previously. The trick is to find the "right balance" that fits you and that you can "live" with!

As stated above, not all calories are created equal. For example, the body is extremely adept at utilizing fat that may be consumed in the diet. In fact, close to 99% of the calories that are derived from fat are capable of being used by the body for energy or being stored as "fat" for future use as energy. We are able to utilize and/or store approximately 96–98% of calories that we consume in the form of carbohydrates. Interestingly, however, we are only able to utilize approximately 78% of calories we consume in the form of proteins. Have you ever felt "warm" after consuming a large steak or other protein rich meal? This was the body's energy necessary to break the "protein bonds" in order to use the energy from the protein itself. While this "taking energy to obtain energy" may seem like a poor use of one's body's reserves, clearly the balance is favorable and the body requires the amino acids that are contained in the proteins in order to stay healthy and repair itself. But beware — too much protein may be as bad as too little.

Diets may result in certain deficiencies with their own health consequences. Kwashiokor is the scientific name of the disease that results from protein deficiency. One does not have to be from a third world country to suffer from this devastating illness — poor people have always tried to make due with what they could afford, often consuming less meat and other protein rich foods that tend to be more costly. Elderly individuals or those who have disabilities may find it hard to obtain fresh food and subsist at times on a diet that has been commonly referred to as the "tea and toast" diet, emphasizing non-perishable food that can be stored at home, especially handy during the cold winter months or when snow or inclement weather make it more difficult to shop. A person with protein deficiency may not at first appear to be "malnourished". In fact, most have an ample layer of subcutaneous fat and may even be obese as they consume plenty of calories, though not enough specific protein. The body requires adequate protein to maintain our immune system, produce necessary enzymes and hormones, and maintain a metabolic balance essential to health. The RDA for protein, or the amount recommended we consume each day, is currently 0.8 grams per kilogram body weight. The weight that should be used in this calculation is "lean weight" as the amount that is calculated is too high if one is obese or fluid filled. While it is recognized that certain individuals may require higher amounts of protein, such as those who lose protein through the GI tract due to an illness, or who are healing from burns or major surgery, data suggest that we might live longer healthier lives if we limited the amount of protein we consume each day to between 0.6 and 0.8 grams per kg body weight, though this currently remains a topic of debate.

Higher levels of ingested protein for prolonged periods may have a negative effect on our kidney function, not over a short period of time, but over a lifetime. In fact, as we age, our kidneys as a product of "normal aging" undergo a 0.6% per year decline in function after age 30. If we believe the data from animal studies, this decline can be accelerated by continued excess protein in the diet as well as by certain diseases that become more common as we age, such as diabetes and hypertension. High dietary protein has been shown in animals to increase the kidney's intraglomerular pressure, setting up a cascade of events that lead to an up-regulation of inflammatory and vasoactive mediators. These result in inflammation and scarring and thus a loss of renal function.

While we all have "extra" kidney function early in life, sufficient to eliminate unwanted products that are filtered through our kidneys, we must not accelerate the normal decline if we are to have sufficient kidney function during our later years. With more people living longer than ever before, prevention is key with this as with all other body components. Excess protein for prolonged periods of time may also cause us to lose bone from our skeleton at a faster rate than we otherwise would. This is a particular problem if excess protein is consumed from animal sources.

Any diet that has as a major component a "high intake of protein" must be looked at carefully and a decision made as to whether this is going to be a "short term" change or something one plans on doing for the "long term". Clearly, if one was to base a diet on protein, total calorie intake tends to be lower especially if one is limiting carbohydrates at the same time and making up the rest of the calories with fat. We just cannot eat as much protein rich food and fat as we can eat food that is rich in carbohydrates.

In addition, remember the energy required to utilize protein? You not only are most likely eating less, you are also utilizing less of the calories you consume. This is a major formula for successful weight loss early on, but once again, likely at a cost if continued over a long period of time. The truth is that studies have shown that despite the quicker weight loss early on, diets based on high protein and fat intake are harder to remain on over time. After 6 months, there is little difference in weight loss for those who chose the high protein–high fat diet as compared to those consuming a well-balanced diet. After two years, those on the high protein–high fat diet tend to be at a disadvantage in terms of weight loss with the additional potential for negative consequences to their lipid profile, bones, and kidneys. While higher protein intake may be useful if one were to embark on an ambitious exercise program that was aimed at building muscle mass, this too must be balanced with total health if continued for long periods of time.

A diet that minimizes carbohydrates while emphasizing protein and fat also makes your body more "acidic". This will have the benefit of reducing your appetite — not bad for weight loss — but will not be as healthy for our bodies in the long term with negative effects on our kidneys and bones. Taken to excess, this metabolic imbalance may lead to unwanted side-effects even in the short term and deaths have been reported in rare circumstances. As mentioned above, diets that emphasize protein while minimizing the intake of carbohydrate also tend to be higher in fat content than similarly caloric, but "well balanced" diets. Why then are there so many testimonials in support of this approach despite the warnings from many medical experts and commissions?

The premise for this diet is largely based on the belief that carbohydrate rich foods have caused us to become an obese nation! There is some truth in this as carbohydrate rich foods are easy to eat in excess and also are the main stimulants to insulin release. Insulin is capable of stimulating our appetite causing us to be hungry and to eat more; it also helps us more efficiently store what we do not need at that moment for future use in the form of fat. While carbohydrates are nature's way of helping us to keep energy for when we may need it, we can easily exceed what is necessary, store the extra calories as fat, and have an excess of unwanted fat. Carbohydrates also lead to a higher circulating level of triglycerides. Fortunately, recent data suggests that this type of elevation of triglycerides in itself and in the absence of an elevation in other "bad" forms of cholesterol (LDL cholesterol) is not as unhealthy as previously thought and clearly less dangerous than the elevated LDL cholesterol that is associated with diets high in fat.

Carbohydrates provide a ready source of utilizable energy, but even here not all carbohydrates are created equal. Some carbohydrates are characterized as "simple" and others as "complex"; some have a high glycemic index, while others have a low glycemic index value. Complex carbohydrates are broken down more slowly by the body and result in a more even level of blood sugar throughout the day and thus are the preferred forms of carbohydrates. It is the "refined" sugars, those that are not the usual form found in nature, that cause the rapid up and down movement of our blood sugar and the wide swings in our insulin levels. Insulin is a hormone that is made in the pancreas and is responsible for taking sugar out of the blood and driving it into the muscles and liver in order to produce energy. Without insulin, we lack the ability to use sugars with the end result being the disease of diabetes mellitus and its resulting high blood sugar and end organ damage. Insulin is essential if we are to lead healthy lives; nevertheless, we can have "too much" insulin as may occur in someone who is obese (large fat cells are more resistant to the action of insulin than normal sized cells). In this case, insulin levels are high throughout the day in an attempt to override the resistance that exists. This is known as "insulin resistance" and may be associated with high blood pressure, increased lipid levels, and high blood sugar levels.

Glycemic Index (GI)

Certain foods are more quickly broken down into sugars and are referred to as having a "high glycemic index". These foods are thought by some to more easily promote weight gain and thus are primary targets in diets that focus on carbohydrate restriction. Many believe that choosing foods with a low glycemic index results in less fluctuation in blood glucose and insulin levels and helps reduce the risk of heart disease and diabetes while promoting weight loss, increasing the body's sensitivity to insulin, reducing hunger, and promoting physical endurance. While data is mixed regarding this approach, in my opinion, avoiding too many portions of foods with a high glycemic index appears to be advantageous at least from a theoretical perspective.

Foods considered to have a low glycemic index have a glycemic score of less than 45; a medium glycemic index is considered to be between 46 and 59; and a high glycemic index is considered to be greater than 60. The following list divides commonly eaten foods by GI. There is some variability among sources as to the GI of various foods but the following is meant as a guide if you choose to use GI in your dietary planning.

Glycemic Index of Commonly Eaten Foods

Grains and Pasta

Low GI: Barley, rice bran, vermicelli, wheat bran, whole rye.

Medium GI: Brown rice, white and wild rice, oatmeal, oat bran, muesli, popcorn, corn, bulgur, rice vermicelli, special K cereal.

High GI: Bagels, corn flakes, English muffins, rice krispies, rice cakes, rye bread, shredded wheat, couscous, cheerios, white flour products.

Beans

Low GI: Black beans, daal, lentils, kidney beans, navy beans, pinto beans, soybeans.

Medium GI: Baked beans, romano beans, chick peas.

High GI: Fava beans.

Dairy

Low GI: Plain yogurt, skim milk, soy milk.

Medium GI: Fruit-flavored low-fat yogurt.

High GI: Low-fat and regular ice cream.

Fruits and Nuts

Low GI: Apple, cherries, dried apricots, nuts, orange, peach, pear, plum, peanuts.

Medium GI: Banana, blueberry, kiwi, mango, orange juice.

High GI: Pineapple, raisins, watermelon.

Vegetables

Low GI: Green beans, peas, tomato, green vegetables, lettuce.

Medium GI: Raw carrots, sweet potatoes, white potatoes (boiled), yams.

High GI: Beets, cooked carrots, mashed potatoes, pumpkin, parsnips, sweet corn.

Depending on your view-point and choice of diet, choosing foods with lower GI may be useful in helping to lower your variations in blood sugar and insulin levels though everything must be taken into consideration as this "fine tuning" of one's diet will be for naught if one does not consider the total calorie intake, choice and amount of fat in the diet, and ingestion of hidden additives all too commonly used in the food production industry such as corn syrup and fructose. I was recently surprised to learn that corn syrup is frequently used in the manufacture of white bread as it helps produce a nice shiny top to the bread and increases the shelf-life of the packaged product. Read labels!

25

Want to Lose Weight?

Helping YOU to Make the Right Diet Choice

There continues to be debate as to what is the "best" diet with believers and non-believers providing testimonials. No one single diet has stood the test of time and clearly there is a need to individualize and choose what will "work" for YOU based on your likes and dislikes, economic factors, and lifestyle. Low carb, no-carb, low fat, no fat are just a few of the themes of various diets. The answer is simple — losing weight demands that one consumes less calories than one utilizes. This "negative calorie balance" is essential and can be achieved through many routes. Not all may work for you or may fit your individual needs. Most diets now focus not just on calories, but how the calories are distributed and how it affects your body's metabolism, most significantly your levels of blood sugar and insulin.

Most diets consist of 30 to 65% carbohydrates. Carbohydrate containing foods provide a rich source of vitamins and minerals, provide dietary fiber and a ready source of energy. Carbohydrates, however, are broken down into small sugar molecules that can be absorbed through the intestine and used by our cells for energy after being converted into glucose. Excess glucose that is formed is stored as fat and leads to weight gain. This process also may stimulate insulin production; while necessary for the uptake and use of glucose by cells in the body, insulin also helps promote fat formation and increases appetite.

In addition, not all carbohydrates are created equally. Complex carbohydrates contain more fiber and are not as easily broken down into sugars. These are often referred to as "good carbs" and should be encouraged as studies have actually demonstrated that complex carbohydrates improve insulin sensitivity at the cellular level and thus may even reduce circulating levels of insulin, a good thing. Fiber has many health benefits as discussed previously. Good carbs come from vegetables, whole grains, and fruits.

Bad carbs are otherwise known as "refined" starches and sugars and include such food as white bread, white pasta, flour, sugar, candy, cookies and most snacks. This form of carbohydrate is quickly broken down into sugar and causes rapid blood sugar swings and thus causes insulin levels to rise dramatically. This "up and down" causes us to have mood swings, become sleepy, and may even result in a feeling of "hyperness" that some have likened to attention deficit syndrome in both adults and children.

Most individuals who eat a diet that is high in carbohydrates take in a higher number of calories than those who eat most of their food as fat and protein. It is much easier to gorge that pasta or to consume many slices of bread, for example, than to eat a plate of meat and high fat foods. Carbohydrates, especially if they are of the "bad" type or that have a "high glycemic" index and are more readily converted into sugar, also raise insulin levels more quickly. The end result is a greater stimulus to eat even more.

Fats and proteins do not have this same effect and in fact cause anorexia if eaten to the exclusion of carbohydrates. Proteins also take more internal energy to digest and thus only 78% of consumed protein is utilized by the body as compared to greater than 95% for both fat and carbohydrates. Both proteins and carbohydrates have 4 calories per gram with fat having 9. It should not be an all or none, however, and you can control what you eat to stay healthy and keep your calories within the desired range. We need to recognize that we need a full complement of nutrients and there are many ways to achieve this goal. Some diet plans work better for an individual than others — the trick is finding something that will have lasting effects and one that will promote wellness and that you can stay with for the long term. Most persons who diet do so for only brief periods, have a variable amount of success, and as time passes, gain the weight back or even more than they lost. Sometimes, they may even have acquired "bad eating habits" and are worse off than when they initially started on the diet.

Particular diets may also have long term consequences. While we now know that diets that are relatively high in fat and protein may help jump-start a diet and result in a greater success in weight reduction early on, these diets appear to lose their advantage after six months and after two years may actually be less helpful than conventional diets that are easier to comply with over time.

Diets may also have unwanted consequences. Most people on a diet rich in protein and fat containing foods begin to add back at least some carbohydrate containing foods as time passes; when this occurs, there is no longer the "acidosis" or change in the chemical composition in the body, and the anorexia, or loss of appetite that occurred with the high fat and protein intake no longer exists. Additionally, diets high in fat and protein may result in problems with bone loss and an accelerated loss of kidney function not to mention setting into place bad habits of eating foods containing high amounts of dietary fat with the many negative health consequences stated previously.

Perhaps one of the most important factors to consider prior to embarking on a diet is to ask the question: Is this a diet I can stick to for a period of time? It is then essential that you become as familiar as possible with the philosophy of the diet, what foods are able to be consumed, and whether it is practical for your lifestyle and other health issues. Financial factors must also be considered as choosing a diet of pre-prepared meals or a diet based on some costly item that you cannot afford to purchase is a set-up for failure. If possible, find others who have been on the specific diet you are evaluating and discuss it with them. Find out what issues came up for them and consider how these might interact with your particular set of circumstances and limitations.

As stated previously, we live in a "fast-food" environment and lead busy, often hectic lives with little time for our own indulgence and pleasure. While we eat to obtain nutrients to remain healthy and frankly, to survive, eating should be a pleasure; but for some, it is something we do without thinking or in response to nervous tension or as a way of distraction. It is amazing just how many calories one can consume without thinking about it or even being aware of what is being ingested. Since it takes a while before the stomach and our organism senses that it is "full" following the ingestion of food, eating more slowly can in itself reduce our calorie intake.

Eating is a social behavior. Persons who have been eating their meals with others in a social context who find themselves suddenly alone, such as after the death of a spouse or after children leave home, often have a reduced intake of food. Add on top of this, a possible depression that may also reduce the desire to eat, one can clearly see how our social structure is the foundation of our diet. These social eating situations may also be responsible for a higher intake of calories with distractions, additional time at the dining table, and perhaps even a greater choice of available foods than one might have when eating alone often responsible for a higher calorie intake.

Before planning a diet, make a list of the characteristics of your eating situation and what factors do you think either tend to increase or decrease your eating tendencies. Do you eat out of frustration or for some secondary gain such as a "release" or to find "comfort"? Many children associate "happy times" with snacks while they sit glued to the TV set or perhaps the time in the day that they can spend with their parents or friends. As we age, these associations become ingrained and become lifelong "habits" that we must deal with head-on. Eating while mindlessly listening to music or talk shows on the radio or watching TV, may mimic this same response and result in a higher calorie intake than otherwise necessary.

As mentioned previously, everyone requires a different amount of calories to maintain their current weight based on what types of food they eat and how they eat them, their body composition, exercise program, and genetic factors that determine how we are able to utilize our consumed calories. Even the number of fat cells we have influences our ability to metabolize foods. Furthermore, it is essential to remember that not all foods are handled the same way in our bodies despite the amount of calories listed on their labels or in a book. Despite this, diets must be structured to ensure that we remain healthy and do not suffer long-term consequences. They must also be structured to allow us to stay on the diet for relatively long periods of time given the reality that weight loss will be a slow process. Rapid changes in weight usually come from a loss of fluid in the body and are transient. Anyone can lose weight through the use of diuretics, though this is a false sense of accomplishment, short-lived, and unhealthy.

Helpful Diet Tips

After establishing your current calorie intake by use of a diet diary, assume that this is the number of calories that is maintaining your weight at its current level. Start to diet by reducing calorie intake by approximately 500 to 1,000 calories a day, depending on how many calories you are starting with and how fast you want to lose weight. You will need to make individual adjustments to keep on your desired path. Remember that your body will "down-regulate" your metabolism upon consuming less calories than it has become accustomed to so you will lose weight in plateaus and may need to continue to fine-tune your diet plan over time. If you have any doubt that you will be able to obtain your necessary vitamins and minerals while dieting, plan on taking a simple daily vitamin and mineral supplement. This is essential for anyone planning to eat less than 1,500 calories a day as your choice of foods will be limited and thus you will more likely be deficient in one or more vitamins and minerals.

Be Consistent

Consistency in your calorie intake will help you to keep on your diet plan. Recognize that you may lose weight at a variable rate so do not weigh yourself too frequently as this may lead to frustration and "burn-out".

Distribute Calories Throughout the Day

Eating three to five times a day (three meals and two low calorie snacks) to provide the target calories you have chosen will produce maximal metabolic effects as compared to eating fewer meals with long periods of starvation in-between. Make sure that the total amount of calories consumed, however, does not increase merely because you are eating more frequently. Remember to drink sufficient amounts of water or low calorie drinks as well. A significant amount of the necessary fluid you take in each day is in the form of "hydrated food"; a diet will reduce your food intake and therefore also your intake of necessary fluid potentially leading to dehydration. This is particularly an issue for the older person who already has less intracellular fluid.

Take Necessary Steps to Manage Stress

Stressful situations should be dealt with prior to starting on a diet if you are to achieve maximal benefit and long-term success; a stress management mechanism should be perfected. It is not uncommon to find individuals during periods of stress, eating more than they otherwise would and perhaps even turning to foods they associated with happier times earlier in their lives. These "comfort foods" may be high calorie foods or snacks and clearly may pre-dispose someone to weight gain. Stress may result in mindless eating! We must not underestimate the interaction between the mind and body even in our consumption of food.

Be Realistic

Once it has been decided that a formal diet is necessary to achieve a particular goal of weight loss, the actual amount of calories to be consumed will need to be determined using a realistic approach. In general, a reduction of 500 calories per day from what someone has been consuming will result in one-half to one pound of weight loss per week in most individuals. If exercise is emphasized, up to 2 pounds is a possibility and within reach. Since we lose weight in stages and reach plateaus along the way, caution is advised to not weigh oneself too frequently as "burn out" becomes a real possibility when weight loss is not continually noted. Keeping to the diet and exercise program, however, will help one achieve long-term goals.

Maintain a Diary

A diary should be started to record weight, body measurements, diet ingested each day or at least at weekly intervals if consistency has been achieved, the type and amount of exercise, and thoughts on the process. It is amazing just how many people have no idea of exactly how many calories they are consuming each day. The better we can document one's dietary intake, the better we can understand why goals may not be achieved and modify the diet in order to achieve these. As each person comes to the table with a unique set of circumstances, body habitus, and biological parameters that will interplay with the chosen diet, flexibility may be necessary in order to achieve the "right" diet for you!

Pay Attention to Portion Size

Knowing what size portion yields how many calories is an essential part of any diet. Some persons prefer a diet that is based on pre-measured and pre-prepared foods to take the guesswork and need for tedious measurements out of one's daily routine. This approach results in a simple way to know exactly how many calories will be contained in the food to be eaten that day. This is not readily possible for all persons due to the often prohibitive cost of purchasing such diets. Limiting the types of food one eats and knowing as much about them as possible, however, including the calorie content for a given amount, is possible and allows each of us to more easily calculate and maintain a given calorie diet.

Avoid Temptation

Whatever diet we eventually choose, carefully define what will be eaten at each meal and place this on your plate prior to coming to the table to remove any temptation or variation. Sharing meals with others is part of our social behavior and must not be avoided; taking food from common serving platters, however, introduces a potentially harmful variable and often leads to greater portion size or servings than are called for in the diet. Remove food from the house that will be an unwanted temptation and substitute it with lower calorie choices.

Eat Mindfully

We need to be Mindful of our eating and be aware of each moment we eat. Mindless eating may cause us to eat quantities of food that are more than necessary and may also make the diet less enjoyable. Prior to starting to eat, take a moment to be appreciative of what is there before you even take your first bite; it may not be what you are used to eating or may appear to be less than you had hoped for but it is the pathway to your new journey of weight loss and a healthier you.

Take a deep breath and exhale slowly to the count of five as you consider how this particular diet and meal will help you achieve your goal of weight reduction. Repeat this process for a few minutes and think positively with an image of your "desired self" clear in mind. Put outside thoughts aside, not blocking them, but allowing them to surface and then let them leave your thoughts, much like a friend who has come to visit but now must go. You can and should return to these thoughts at a later time after the meal is over.

As described in more detail in the chapter on Mind/Body, appreciate the many colors, textures, and tastes as you slowly ingest each bite. Upon completing the meal, spend a few minutes and remain mindful of your goals and the process that will take you to them. Finish again with your desired image in mind and breathe deeply, exhaling to the count of five, and repeating this between five and ten times prior to excusing yourself from the dining table.

With time, this process will become second nature and you will learn to incorporate the process of Eating Mindfully to each meal and hopefully through this, not only enjoy your meals to a greater degree, but eat in a more healthy manner.

CHAPTER

26

Final Considerations Prior to Choosing the "Right" Diet for YOU

While we are all aware of studies linking high fat diets to diseases including cardiovascular disease and certain cancers such as breast, prostate, and colon, a certain amount of fat in the diet is essential for the maintenance of our nervous system. While Eskimos and other arctic region dwellers consume large quantities of fat in their diet, it is not something we want others to do. Since fat contains 9 calories in every gram as compared to 4 for carbohydrate and protein it is a very efficient source of energy and a way of meeting high calorie demands when you are stranded in the arctic and have to make it through those cold winter nights. For the rest of us, however, fat should never exceed 30% of our total calorie intake with lower amounts suggested for those with a high risk of developing heart disease or who already have it. Unfortunately, the average American woman consumes 39% of their diet as fat, raising calorie intake, promoting obesity, and increasing the risk of disease.

As noted previously in this book, not all fats are created equal. There is saturated fat and unsaturated fat. Unsaturated fat is further divided into polyunsaturated or monounsaturated. Animal derived fat is saturated and has the most health risks associated with it including a risk of certain cancers and heart disease. Not all fat derived from vegetables is as healthy as many believe. Coconut and palm oil, major fats used in the preparation of packaged cookies and cakes due to their low cost, consist largely of saturated fats. Olive oil and canola oil are both largely monounsaturated fats and are considered to be the healthiest, but here again only if consumed in moderation. How about corn or safflower oil? These are derived from vegetables and are polyunsaturated when in the oil form. If made into a solid such as margarine, however, they become saturated during the production process. It is for this reason that we often get confused when we buy a vegetable margarine thinking it is all polyunsaturated when in fact we are getting "trans fats" or "hydrogenated oils". Some have argued that these artificially produced fats are even more unhealthy than saturated fats themselves. This message became even clearer to me when I noted in a popular health food store that their brand of organic peanut butter contained added palm oil, apparently to create a more "appealing" product to the consumer. It was listed as an ingredient in small print but I am certain most people thought they were buying the "real thing" when they purchased their product in the health food store under the organic label. Buyers beware as not everything labeled as organic is as healthy as you might be led to believe!

Once again, I return to the problem of portion size. I am sure you have been to the Italian restaurant and were impressed by the fact that the warm freshly made bread came not with pats of butter or margarine, but rather seasoned olive oil. How quickly the bread soaked up the oil equivalent to multiple pats of butter or margarine. For an equivalent amount of fat, you would have been better off with the oil; however, when taken to excess, even monounsaturated fats have their downside — all it takes is a conscious effort and common sense to eat healthy.

Fiber was mentioned previously as a necessary component of a healthy diet and an excellent way of helping to prevent many diseases included colon cancer, diverticulosis, gallbladder disease, hemorrhoids, and even hypercholesterolemia. Certain fibers have also been shown to have a positive effect on our metabolic state and blood glucose control. The trick is just how to consume the 30 grams of fiber each day that has been associated with the greatest impact on one's health in numerous world-wide studies. At least one-third of the daily fiber intake should be in the form of a soluble fiber with the remaining coming from foods rich in insoluble fibers. This is essential if we are to achieve maximum benefit. In recent years there has been talk that fiber is not as beneficial as it was previously thought to be. This conclusion was made following the analysis of a large population based study of American nurses. The study population was divided into five groups, or quintiles. When the "top" quintile was compared to the "lowest" in terms of fiber intake and correlated with associated disease, there was little difference in at least one measure, e.g. colon cancer recurrence. No mention was made of the many other possible benefits of sufficient fiber in the diet. If one analyzed the study further, however, one noted that even the group consuming the most fiber took in only approximately 20 grams of fiber, not the 30 grams thought to be necessary for optimal benefit as demonstrated in international studies using populations that consume on average a great deal more fiber as part of their natural diet.

Many foods have been found to have beneficial effects if taken in moderation despite their caloric content and even relatively high amount of fat. Nuts are one such example. An excellent source of fiber and protein, nuts contain high amounts of monounsaturated fats with almonds and walnuts being particularly useful as noted earlier in this book. Dark chocolate is another example of a food that is commonly thought of as being a poor diet choice; if taken in moderation, however, there is some evidence that it may actually have a beneficial effect on one's "good" form of cholesterol (HDL) and may also reduce cardiovascular risk by causing our platelets to be less "sticky" and therefore reducing their chances of clumping together and causing heart attacks. Dark chocolate in moderation may also reduce inflammation that has been linked to heart disease and frailty later in life. Consuming a modest amount of red wine or red grape juice may also have benefit though clearly alcohol consumption has its own set of risks to consider. The skin of the red grape contains resveratrol, an antioxidant and studies suggest a possible beneficial effect on reducing cardiovascular disease and even the risk of developing lung cancer.

In searching for the optimal diet, I was continually intrigued by a wealth of data regarding specific foods that have been shown to have potential benefit to one's health. I came to the conclusion, however, that many diets can yield benefit if considered in the context of their own strengths and weaknesses and continued over time. A lifetime of health, however, may not be compatible with a particular diet, especially if it yields only a short-term commitment on your part or does not provide you with a well-balanced choice of foods.

There is no shortage of diets to choose from and you may find something that stimulates interest at every turn; remember that choosing the "right" diet is not an easy task and the choice must not be taken lightly as it will lead you down a path that may help you reach your diet goals but also may have health consequences. A diet that is based on scientific evidence with proven benefit should be the goal for us all. Data are not always available or reliable and the impact that a diet has long-term on one's health is usually not something discussed. Which diet will work for a given person is a very individual choice. Almost any diet, if done correctly has the potential to help you lose undesirable weight, but for how long and at what risk?

There has been success with diets that limit the choice of foods to only a few, even if they are not in themselves of any special value in terms of health consequences. Once again, it is all about one's ability to comply with the diet and calorie restriction and the long-term health consequences of the nutrients we eat or fail to eat for prolonged periods of time.

Weight Watchers has proven to have great long term success for those who continue with the diet plan, though many believe that this is due to the psychological effects from the meetings that take place with "peer pressure" or maybe even humiliation as motivating factors. Weight Watchers as a company has also developed its own product line with calorie restricted portions that have been assigned "points" for comparison and substitution ability. These are available for purchase in most supermarkets and if one so chooses can help take out the guesswork as to calories and food choices.

For some, a dramatic "jump start" may be the only way to begin the life changing process. This may produce more rapid results and help increase one's motivation to stay the course. This form of diet, however, is usually not appropriate for maintenance due to some component that may be either excessive or deficient if continued for too long. In this case, the individual is faced with a new diet and may gain back whatever weight was lost as part of the initial "jump start" process. Many "jump start" diet programs are also based on a repetitive diet that becomes increasingly difficult to comply with. It is also important to remember that this method of dieting fails to provide a strategy for long-term benefit and must be coupled with a more comprehensive diet plan if one is to be successful meeting specific goals over time.

For individuals who are extremely well motivated and who feel they can control their urges, a more gentle and well balanced approach may be the way to go and in fact may lead to improved dietary habits in short order that can have more long-lasting benefit and promote a more healthy state throughout life.

Clearly the quantity of weight one wishes to lose and one's underlying health status are key to what diet is "best" for any individual. A medical clearance may also be necessary especially for those with underlying medical illness, the elderly, or those seeking to loose more than 10% of their weight. An exercise regimen must be integrated into any diet plan to achieve maximal benefit and life long success. A daily vitamin is also suggested for anyone who is not continuing to consume a well-balanced diet or who is eating less than 1,500 calories a day; at this level, there simply is too restrictive a choice of foods to ensure optimal nutrient intake. By a daily vitamin, I am referring to a simple combination vitamin and mineral complex available at any pharmacy or supermarket and not a "mega-vitamin" or individual vitamins of large quantities. Read labels carefully to find the proper vitamin, usually a generic brand that provides basic requirements and may also provide certain nutrients such as antioxidants. The most expensive vitamin you can buy is not necessarily better in my opinion. Be a smart consumer and know what you are buying! Be cautious as well of bargain basement deals available at discount stores or on-line as purity and the risk of contamination with other undesirable contents remain variables to consider.

There are few regulations on the health food industry and I have seen patients become toxic from products that were not manufactured with skill in mind. One patient of mine became toxic from Vitamin A when they thought they were taking only Vitamin D; both are fat soluble vitamins and the purification process used in the manufacture of the product this person was taking was clearly not sufficient to prevent contamination. I also have seen a tragic case of a young boy who prematurely stopped growing due to the closure of his bone growth plates. After a very exhaustive search, it was uncovered that this boy had been taking daily vitamins that were bought in a foreign country when his family went on vacation. Although these vitamins were cheap and thus the reason the family bought large quantities of them, they contained various hormones known to restrict growth — a tragic story that I will never forget.

Diets come in a variety of types and each contains a range of calories. The trick is to determine what will work for YOU! While a deficit of 3,500 calories represents approximately one pound potentially lost, at least theoretically, due to the way each of us handles the calories we eat each day, and depending on what you eat, it may or may not result in the loss of one pound and you must not be disappointed if there is not an immediate drop in weight. Remember, our bodies strive to keep us in balance with our existing weight and we must re-adjust our metabolism in order to begin the weight reduction process. Weight is also a composite of many body components including water, fat, and muscle. The goal is to lose fat while maintaining or even building muscle mass. Most acute weight loss comes from the loss of water in the body, a short lived effect that is not the goal of any weight loss program.

There is a great deal of variability from person to person as to just how successful our diets will be so be patient and remember that you will likely need to individualize a diet just with you in mind. This may take time and patience is necessary to avoid "burn out". People who are overweight tend to be more "efficient" in handling their calories and can drop their calories at times quite significantly and still see no immediate weight loss. Keeping to the plan and staying the course will yield eventual benefit.

As mentioned previously, any combination of diet and exercise program that causes us to utilize more calories than we consume will result in "some" weight loss over time. Pick a number, begin the process and adjust as you see what is happening to you. Keep a diary to record what you are eating, your changing body measurements, and weight, but do not become consumed by the process — expect to see plateaus and even some up and down shifts as the body re-adjusts to the new diet, has shifts in fluid, and other natural variations take place. Even the menstrual cycle may influence your results with accumulation of fluid by the body masking weight loss. If you do not get the results you want after the first few weeks, it is time to re-evaluate. You can always increase your activity, walk an extra mile, jog for a few extra minutes each day, swim an extra lap, or whatever routine gives you pleasure and burns those unwanted calories. Similarly, you can adjust your dietary intake — increase or decrease your calories — to achieve the end result you desire.

27

Ten Helpful Suggestions to Help YOU Lose Unwanted Weight and Keep It Off!

The following are suggestions that may help YOU make the right choices as you embark on a diet that you can live with and that will help you to achieve a successful aging process. Many persons who choose to follow the simple suggestions listed below will lose unwanted weight. Just how much will depend on your own circumstances but at least you will be ahead of the game and any further weight loss you desire can be achieved with these health promoting principles to build upon. These suggestions will also sustain you as you seek to maintain your accomplishments and continue to promote optimal health throughout your life.

Whatever path you choose, it must be carefully designed to not only produce weight loss if this is a goal, but to provide you with a framework upon which to improve your health status and quality of life for the long-term. It must be a diet you can live with even after you achieve your goals and that allows you to continue to enjoy life's many pleasures.

1. **Become knowledgeable!**
   Reading books such as this one can help you to better understand your choices; choose foods and methods of food preparation that may help you to achieve optimal health. Know which foods to avoid.

2. **Make goals for yourself!**
   Make goals that include both short-term and long-term objectives. How fast do you want to achieve your goals and how much are you willing to

"change" your daily routine to accomplish them? Is the diet plan you are considering one that you believe you can remain on or is this only a means to a quick goal? Know what you can expect!

3. **Make an inventory of what you are doing NOW!**
Keeping a diary for two to three weeks prior to embarking on your life-changing plan will likely provide you with new insights into "why" you are in the situation you are in. You hopefully will be able to review this diary with someone knowledgeable such as your physician or a dietitian or after doing some more reading. By understanding your own eating habits, food choices, portion size, how you prepare your food, amount, duration and type of exercise, and other aspects of your daily life you will most likely increase your awareness of what you will need to do to change.

It is amazing just how many people do not stop to consider the calories of the three cans of soda they drink each day or the fruit juice they were substituting for previously consumed soda thinking it was "healthy" and therefore not necessary to account for. When considering portion size, it is not only necessary to consider this for the main source of protein, such as meat, fish, or poultry, but also for the side dishes such as rice, noodles, or potatoes. The amount and type of salad dressing added to a low calorie salad is another area that often escapes recognition but can add a significant number of unnecessary calories.

I had a patient who was having a hard time losing weight. The diet seemed appropriate and I had seen some progress over time but it had slowed and now he found himself on a plateau for too long. Upon careful questioning I was able to uncover that my patient had started eating "diet cookies" about the time of the change in progress. He bought these after reading the word "diet" on the label on the box and thought that these would "promote weight loss" in some unknown manner. I needed to educate him that in this case, "diet" referred to the smaller size of the cookie and its relatively fewer calories as compared to a more normally sized product. These "diet cookies" however, also had calories to be considered and the more he ate of these, the harder it would be to maintain his planned calorie intake despite his thinking that "more was good" as a way to promote his desired weight loss.

4. **Determine what plan of action you believe will be best for YOU!**
Do you want to see "big" results fast or are you willing to see "slow progress"? Are you willing to change your daily routine dramatically to achieve your goals or do you prefer to do your best to incorporate slow changes into your current lifestyle realizing that the changes will take longer to achieve? Be realistic, but remain positive!

5. **Remember the Mind/Body Connection!**
    Remember that our body is connected to our mind and the mind/body connection is a potent one that may prove harmful or helpful depending on how you use it! Make a list of daily stressors in your life, adding a section in your diary for this purpose. Perhaps list those issues that remain as challenges to your mental health and give thought to how you might resolve these both in the short and long term and who you will need to work with to accomplish your goals. Seek help as appropriate whether it involves "talking" to your physician, a clergy member, a psychologist, a psychiatric social worker, friend or family member. Remember that Mindfulness Training and the use of other mind/body techniques as listed previously in this book may be necessary and something you need to embark on even before you begin your diet and exercise plan. Resolving underlying issues that create stress and anxiety should be a top priority not only to help ensure success with your diet and exercise program but also to help you age more successfully! Approach all of your daily activities in a more "Mindful" manner and remember to Eat Mindfully!

6. **Determine what is a "Deal Breaker"!**
    Determine what is a "Deal Breaker" to you and commit it to writing. By this I mean, list any strong likes or dislikes that you feel are impossible to surmount either in terms of time, activity, or diet. If you just cannot find the time to go to a gym to exercise, for example, there is no need for you to plan on this activity as your basis of increasing your level of physical activity — you will need to find an alternate way to exercise to meet your goals. If you are required to eat or not eat certain foods or nutrients or have strong food preferences, you would be wise to choose a diet that will allow you to live within your limitations rather than use some pre-determined diet that violates your desires and exceeds your boundaries of tolerability.

7. **How flexible are you?**
    Are you willing to try new things or are you fairly "fixed in your ways"? Make a list of the last 5 "new" things you were willing to try. How successful were you in doing them? Rate the success on a scale of 1 being "not very successful" and 5 being "totally successful". Where are you on average? This may help you to decide just how "adventurous" you are willing to be. If your average score is less than 3, for example, you will likely be more successful in trying to modify your daily routine more slowly, perhaps making one change a week and not introducing another one until you feel that you have reached your short term goal.

8. **Determine how fast you want to see results.**
    Depending on how fast you want to see results, you may choose an alternate diet plan. If you want to see results more quickly, you may be

tempted to try to "Jump Start" your "new self". While this may not be what the "doctor ordered" for everyone, those who think they may benefit from something that will yield quicker results as a means of motivation or for some other personal reason, may find this a useful approach. Even if only to demonstrate to yourself that "change is possible", this approach will allow you to think "differently". Whether it is a plan for a weekend, a week, or even one month, a change that breaks your "old traditions" and establishes that a new phase of your life is beginning may "jump start" you and yield positive results. Remember that this will not be a long-term approach either for weight loss or health promotion and that "quick weight loss" diets usually lead to weight gain later on. Repeating this process frequently with fluctuations in weight will in itself have negative effects on one's health. Only embark on this approach if it is part of a larger diet plan that you expect to continue.

9. **Seek Support in Advance of Starting Something New!**
   Even before you begin your life-changing path, seek support from family and friends. Having an intricate diet and exercise plan is for naught if you are surrounded with temptations at every turn and competing interests. Enter into frank discussions as to your planned activities that are needed if you are to accomplish your goals and let others know what you expect of them. Ask for periodic feedback and let them know that their encouragement is greatly appreciated as you enter into what will most likely be a very challenging time in your life. While your diet is a very personal choice, it may also impact on others and it is wise to consider just how this may play out before problems occur either for you or your loved ones.

10. **Put yourself first!**
    This time is ALL about YOU. Rewards from the positive changes that take place will pay back others in spades.

CHAPTER

28

Dieting: What Are My Choices?

As mentioned previously, any weight loss program that you choose to embark upon must be individually planned and something that "fits" with your lifestyle. It must not exceed your financial limitations and ideally will yield long term results. When choosing your diet plan, make sure that it can help you achieve not only your goal of weight loss, but also promote optimal health! It must provide you with a framework upon which to help you select, prepare, and eat healthy foods while also providing you with an exercise program that will allow you to increase your activity, build muscle mass, and improve your endurance level. While increasing one's exercise throughout the day will add up and help one achieve certain goals, a regimen that provides a minimum of 30 minutes of vigorous exercise at least three times each week yields greater benefit to cardio-vascular health and is encouraged if possible. Additional time exercising will help one to burn additional calories and help build muscle though even here, more is not always better and too much exercise of certain types can lead to muscle tears, limited recovery time, and strains, sprains, and pain!

Diet programs that promise immediate weight loss and do not have a maintenance plan built into them, are more risky and in my opinion less likely to succeed in helping you to achieve your lifelong goals over the long haul. There are fad diets advertised almost every month, some gaining a great deal of popularity, but few stand the test of time and meet healthy nutritional goals. You may have heard of some of them such as the Grapefruit Diet, The Rice Diet, the Cabbage Soup Diet, the No Carbs Diet, the Low Fat Diet, and many others.

I have tried to provide you with a framework in this book to help you appreciate that we require a well balanced diet for maximal long-term health and as successful an aging process as possible. For most persons, eating a healthy mix of foods does not in itself lead to weight gain; the problem comes when there is a poor choice of food or food preparation, an excessive quantity of calories consumed, and/or a lack of sufficient exercise to help with metabolism. Exercise alone, however, will not be sufficient for most persons wishing to lose more than a modest amount of weight. Starting an exercise program alone will help one lose on average 6–8 pounds while the average diet helps one lose on average 20 pounds. It is important to remember, however, that this is an average value and that the weight following exercise may be misleading due to the greater amount of muscle that weighs more than the fat it replaces. To lose one pound per week through exercise alone, however, the average person would need to walk in excess of 5 miles per day every day of the week or some other equivalent exercise regimen. A combination of diet and exercise remains the best option for a healthy and viable plan.

The Following is an Attempt to Summarize to the Best of My Ability My Thoughts Regarding Several of the More Popular Diets that have been Proposed in Recent Times

Body-for-Life

This diet is a three month program that is based on eating a diet high in protein combined with a regular exercise regimen. While it suggests that one eat six meals a day with an emphasis on portion size, it does not regulate the amount of calories consumed. Each meal is to include one portion of protein and one portion of carbohydrate; a vegetable is added to two of the meals. Each week one is allowed to eat a more unrestricted diet for a day. This diet is limited in variety and does not strive to provide all of the nutrients required for lifelong health.

Low Fat

Dean Ornish, MD has touted this form of diet that combines vegetarian and low-fat meals to achieve its results. While there is data to suggest that the very low 10% fat intake promotes a healthy heart, slowing or in some cases even reversing coronary artery disease, it is restrictive in its content in terms of variety and many find it difficult to continue over time. The diet plan also encourages daily exercise.

The American Heart Association has also supported a low-fat, restricted calorie diet with no more than 30% of calories derived from fat (10% from saturated fat) and no more than 300 mg cholesterol daily. This diet is largely based on a diet rich in low-fat grains, vegetables, fruits and legumes with restrictions on adding additional fat and sweets. A carefully planned Mediterranean Diet will meet this criteria.

Healthy Weight Pyramid

This diet was developed at the Mayo Clinic and is based on eating foods that are low-calorie yet energy-dense such as fruits and vegetables. These tend to be large volume foods that help promote a feeling of fullness yet provide fewer calories than customary diets. Daily exercise is encouraged.

Mediterranean Diet

This diet provides a moderate-fat, restricted-calorie regimen that is rich in vegetables and low in red meat. Poultry and fish are staples in this diet. While fat content is generally in the 30–35% range, it promotes the use of olive oil, canola oil, flax seeds, and nuts. Epidemiological studies do support that this diet promotes cardiovascular health, lower lipid values, and reduced rates of constipation, diverticulosis, gall bladder disease, and hemorrhoids due to its relatively high fiber content.

In 1999, the Lyon Diet Heart Study provided evidence that within four years, individuals placed on a standard Mediterranean Diet had reduced their rates of heart disease recurrence and cardiac death by 50 to 70% as compared to individuals placed on a conventional diet offered at that time by the American Heart Association. Since this time, several subsequent studies have confirmed the benefits of this diet. In 2004, a study in Greece evaluated its impact on 3,000 men and women. The diet was associated with improved markers of inflammation and coagulation including C-reactive protein and fibrinogen. A study conducted in the Netherlands reported a 50% lower rate of death from heart disease and from all causes among men and women aged 70 to 90 who followed a Mediterranean diet. These individuals, however, also exhibited other beneficial health practices such as exercising and non-smoking.

Another study evaluated approximately 1,400 individuals without cognitive deficit and 500 with mild cognitive impairment with a mean age of 77 in order to determine the effect of diet on cognition. After nearly five years of follow up, individuals who closely adhered to the principles of a Mediterranean diet had a 28% lower risk of developing mild cognitive impairment compared to those eating a diet not compatible with these principles. While those who partially followed the principles of a Mediterranean diet had a 17% lower risk of developing cognitive impairment than those who did not, this finding failed to reach statistical significance. Of note, eating a Mediterranean diet also appeared to slow down the progression of cognitive decline even after it was diagnosed. There was a 48% lower risk of being diagnosed with Alzheimer's Disease within 4 years among the individuals who were already diagnosed with mild cognitive impairment at the start of the study and who adhered strictly to the Mediterranean diet as compared to those with impairment who did not. The risk was 45% lower for those who at least ate a moderate version of the diet. It was not possible from the study data to determine just how long those individuals who ate a Mediterranean diet were on it prior to entering the study and whether this might have influenced the data. Thus we do not know from this study just how long someone must modify their diet in order to see such dramatic and positive results. We also do not know if these individuals had other behaviors that might have influenced the results; additional research is clearly warranted.

When these and other studies are taken together, there appears to be a great deal of evidence that a diet based on the principles of the Mediterranean diet may offer dramatic benefits in both physical and mental health.

Liquid Meal Combinations

Often referred to as the Slim-Fast Diet after the product with this name, it can be modified to use any brand of available liquid nutrient. This diet is based on consuming liquid shakes for breakfast and lunch, a "reasonable" dinner, and three snacks per day with some modification based on who you read. Two fruit snacks and one pre-packaged snack, initially a Slim-Fast snack bar, was included as part of the daily meal plan. Exercise was also encouraged. This diet clearly requires a repetitive choice of foods and shakes that may not be palatable or provide a full feeling for some. Those who are able to adhere to the repetitive regimen, however, may be able to continue to lose weight and improve various parameters of health such as blood sugar and blood cholesterol.

While Slim-Fast is often chosen as the "shake" for breakfast and lunch, any product such as Carnation Instant Breakfast, Ensure, Sustecal, among others that provide a well balanced meal of approximately 1 calorie per milliliter consumed can be used. While there is some risk in allowing the dieter to plan their own dinner, hopefully the choice of foods will be carefully considered with specific goals and knowledge in mind.

In certain cases based on an individual's unique set of circumstances and needs, I have prescribed a "jump start" diet based on 5 cans of a liquid meal, each providing a well balanced 240 calories spread throughout the day with a multi-vitamin added to ensure adequate nutrition. To this, I advised that 6–8, 8 ounce glasses of water or club soda be consumed and as much salad as is desired be eaten with a low-salt soy sauce and/or vinegar and lemon dressing as a healthy and fiber containing snack. Realizing that this type of a diet will become more difficult to adhere to over time, it must be part of a bigger diet plan. Clearly it will take the guess-work out of eating early in the diet process and may "jump start" your diet with often dramatic results. It clearly is not my suggestion for most persons looking for a proper diet that they can consume long-term. Lack of fiber if a salad is not eaten and once again the limited choice of foods and consistency makes this an extremely difficult diet to remain on for long-term success and health.

Low-Energy-Density Diet

This diet is based on foods that are low in fat and high in fiber. The premise is that these foods will better "fill" the stomach and reduce the feeling of hunger and urge to eat. It relies on the dieter choosing foods that they feel meet this criteria and may be inadequate in certain nutrients if maintained for long periods of time. Whole grains and vegetables are eaten in ample quantity.

Low Carbohydrate Diet

There have been many who claim to have cornered the market on this type of plan. The idea is to limit carbohydrates and thus lower insulin levels and hopefully one's hunger. While some allow carbohydrates to be consumed at one meal each day, the theme is based on limiting the amount of fruit, cereal, breads, pasta, rice, potatoes, etc. This unfortunately limits the amount of fiber one consumes and also tends to promote a higher intake of fat and protein in the diet with negative consequences if consumed for more than a brief period of time. Many feel that persons on this form of diet need not have a pre-determined restriction of calories, being confident that restricting carbohydrates to a maximum of 20 grams per day initially will in itself promote weight loss. While some persons on this diet have carbohydrate intakes as low as 13 grams/day, most feel that any amount below 50 grams/day will lead to ketosis with the result being an acidotic state that promotes anorexia or reduced hunger. Many people on this diet eat fewer calories than one might think; given the choice of foods that are largely fat and protein, most individuals do not replace the lost carbohydrates on a one-to-one basis. Some studies have reported faster loss of weight on this form of diet though this is not universally accepted. Most agree that long term success is less likely and negative health consequences may exceed benefit over time. Given the choice of foods that consist mostly of fat and protein, one must be concerned about accelerating the normal age-related change in kidney function that may result from an excessive intake of protein in the diet and the development of osteoporosis from increased bone turnover. Most suggest that individuals on this form of diet choose vegetarian sources of fat and protein to maximize their nutrient intake.

Blood Type Diet

Dr. D'Adamo claims that depending on your blood type, you will have unique needs and do better with certain foods that he lists in his popular selling book. No scientific data is available to my knowledge to prove that this hypothesis is worth pursuing.

High Fat/High Protein Diet

Popularly referred to as the Atkins' Diet, this diet is similar to the Low Carbohydrate Diet listed above though it reduces carbohydrate intake even further. It allows one to eat protein and fat. As the body burns calories to live, it metabolizes fat and thus promotes an acidosis with its associated anorexia or reduced desire to eat. Since insulin tends to also be lower in the absence of carbohydrate intake, it provides less of a stimulus for us to eat. Clearly the high protein intake helps promote weight loss as there are fewer calories available to the body due to the added energy required to metabolize protein; additionally most persons also eat fewer calories given the limited choice of tempting foods. Increased risk of an accelerated decline in kidney function and a greater tendency of bone turnover leading to osteoporosis are concerns. The high fat diet is also worrisome and over time, the advantages of the quicker weight loss that may result in the early stages of this diet appear to be overshadowed. In addition, many persons are unable or unwilling to continue this diet over the long term and thus begin to modify the choice of foods with time; adding carbohydrates further eliminates the potential benefit and possible reason for its mode of action in the first place.

Revolutionary Weight Control Program

This diet was popularized by Bob Arnot, MD. The diet attempts to teach what order and at what times of day certain foods should be eaten to maximally control weight, mood, and hunger. In general, this diet limits carbohydrates.

Sugar Busters

This diet is based on limiting the intake of refined and processed forms of sugar in the diet such as potatoes, white rice, corn, white bread, carrots, corn syrup, etc. It tends to be high in protein and fat and thus has similar concerns as raised above in similarly structured diets.

The Zone

This diet was popularized by Barry Sears, Ph.D and is based on someone entering "The Zone". To do so, one must eat the "right" amounts of food in "macronutrient blocks" at certain times throughout the day. Carbohydrates, proteins and fats are eaten in a ratio of 40%, 30%, and 30%, respectively. The limited calorie content, in many cases less than 1,000 calories daily, prevents consumption of sufficient nutrients for long term health though it will clearly promote weight loss for those who are compliant.

Soup Diet

Since many people fall off their diets when given too much of a "choice" of what they should eat, eating the same foods day after day takes away a significant risk of non-compliance though risks "burn-out". Many argue that a short period of eating only soup, perhaps no more than one week, can help "jump start" a diet and may even promote faster weight loss. Soups tend to be quite low in calories if one steers clear from cream based soup; some vegetables such as cabbage and leeks reportedly have a mild diuretic effect that helps one to lose weight faster than one otherwise would, though this additional benefit to weight loss is due to a loss of body fluid and will be quickly regained over time. This form of diet clearly places one at risk of failing to obtain proper well balanced nutrition and does nothing to help one learn lifelong proper eating habits. Some individuals complain of ill effects from eating only vegetable based soup due largely to the relatively low calories being consumed and bloating that may result from high amounts of fiber. Depending on the choice of soup, and how it is prepared, however, fiber and other essential nutrients can be obtained. High salt content is often a risk though this can be managed by the use of tasty herbs and spices to help limit the need for salt and carefully selecting low salt soups if one chooses to buy commercially available products.

Having a vegetable or bean-based soup for one meal a day, however, is something to consider as part of any diet as most soups, unless they are cream-based, tend to be lower calorie meals that provide nutrients and often satisfying results regardless of how much one consumes. Adding a green salad, with caution regarding the salad dressing that is added, helps curb appetite even further, provides fiber, and may be used to complement almost any diet. Soups rich in pasta and meats must be considered separately and evaluated as to their calorie and nutrient value as these may defeat your purpose.

Commercial Weight-Loss Programs

There are many weight-loss programs that offer pre-packaged food that takes the guess work out of dieting. Simply decide on the number of calories and combination of meals and snacks, and the rest is left up to the program. The relatively high cost involved and practicality of obtaining the meals may be limiting factors to many persons. Many of these programs combine professional and group session support such as Weight Watchers. The Weight Watchers Program is additionally based on a point system that allows substitution of food choices with a total point goal individually designed for the dieter. Those who are able to stay on such programs can lose weight and studies have shown long term success as well though compliance remains an issue for some.

Very Low Calorie Diets

Diets that limit one intake to less than 800 calories per day lead to more rapid weight loss but should not be used unless there is a particular reason for doing so as the risk of significant muscle loss, electrolyte abnormalities, fatty infiltration of the liver, and other problems are great. Medical supervision is strongly urged if you decide to embark on such a drastic approach. The ability to stay on such a diet is also questionable without significant resources and motivation. Weight-loss required prior to mandatory surgery is one example for being on such a restrictive diet. In general, most persons on this type of diet rely on pre-packaged diet bars, liquid meals, and pre-packaged entrees. The unrestricted use of salads with vinegar and lemon/soy sauce dressing can help provide fiber and help maintain a sense of fullness. Fluids must be encouraged as well as approximately 50% of the fluid we take in each day comes not from what we drink but from the hydration in our solid foods. This diet is so restrictive that fluid deficits are likely without special consideration and added fluid intake. Also remember that weight-loss will initially largely be from a loss of muscle mass unless an exercise program is incorporated; even here, a lack of appropriate nutrients due to the significant calorie restriction may interfere with proper muscle development.

29

The *Be Fit for Life Diet*: A Diet YOU Can Live With

As mentioned several times in this book, a diet that incorporates a well balanced variety of foods to provide protein, carbohydrate and yes, even fat, will yield health benefits if structured correctly. It should be high in complex forms of carbohydrate, contain an adequate amount of soluble and insoluble fiber, have sufficient vitamins, minerals, and anti-oxidants, and limit the amount of protein and fat to acceptable ranges. Perhaps equally as important to knowing what foods to choose as part of a healthy diet is focusing your attention on ways you can modify the way you eat. If done correctly, many persons are surprised to learn that no special diet may be necessary to achieve the goal of a healthier you!

Yes, weight gain and loss is all about the balance between the amount of calories one eats and the calories that you are able to "burn" or metabolize. Health consequences from our diet, however, are more than just the number of calories we eat and burn. We will all need to adjust our diets as we age in order to insure an intake of health promoting nutrients and keep our weight appropriate for our age, height, and body type. Most individuals do have a change in their metabolism and body composition and require fewer calories merely to keep their weight constant with increasing age. This is a simple fact of life and something we must accept and even prepare for!

The following are some practical suggestions that can be incorporated into one's everyday life with very little effort and may be all that is needed to get you on the right path to achieve your goal of life-long health and a more successful aging process. Since some people may require a more limited and defined approach to their individual weight plan, I have included one such diet below that is based on the premise of choosing the most health promoting foods and weight management strategies.

Be Fit for Life Diet Strategy

1. *Practice Mindful Eating*

Recognizing that we often are not even aware of what and how much we are eating at each meal, make a concerted effort to consider each and every food choice and whether "you are sure" this is what you want to eat. Use Mindful Eating to slow you down, increase your enjoyment, and as a tool for weight management.

2. *Consider Spreading Your Calories Throughout the Day*

Remember that for the same amount of calories consumed throughout the day, the "nibbler" or person who spreads these calories into 5 or more meals, will find it easier to eventually lose weight as compared to a person who "binges" or "gorges" themselves with only one or two meals a day with long periods of "fasting" between. The body senses that there are long periods without food and assumes a protective stance by decreasing metabolism. We are shaped not only by "what we eat" but also "how we eat"! While there is a risk of consuming more calories when eating more frequently, a well planned diet that takes the same amount of calories but ensures that they are distributed may help increase metabolism and promote weight loss. If you are a person who eats one large meal and skips others throughout the day, merely changing your pattern of eating may help you to loose weight.

3. *Consider Alternate Choices for Commonly Eaten Foods*

Certain foods will help promote unhealthy dietary habits, increase your appetite, or lead to greater weight gain. These foods are best avoided. Using your diary, record what foods you need to eliminate from your diet and eliminate them from your life. If you are a person who enjoys a "snack" at a certain time of the day, only have those foods available that you have decided are okay to eat. Clean out your pantries and refrigerator and yes, get everyone at home or in the office "on-board"; this is essential for maximal benefit. Carrot sticks, celery, cucumber slices, apples, oranges, and lettuce are excellent low calorie snacks to keep on hand.

4. *Learn to Eat "Frugally"!*

Just as you try to do with your finances, eat frugally and consider your options at all meals. Change the way you eat and what you eat and always consider substitutions that may be more advantageous to you. Refer back to your diary and remember the foods that you consider "comfort foods". Distinguish these from your "everyday foods" and if you are not able to eliminate these completely from your diet, limit eating these foods to one day a week.

5. *Eliminate Added Sugar to Your Coffee, Tea, Cereal, or Fruit*

6. *Artificial Sweeteners Need To Go*

While perhaps providing a pleasurable taste for some, these will only help maintain your addiction to sweets. Break the cycle now. You will soon recognize a change in your food seeking behaviors and stop craving that slice of cake, candy bar, soda, or other high calorie and unhealthy food.

7. *Stop Eating "White Foods" Except Low Fat Dairy Products*

White bread, white rice, white potatoes, and white pasta consist largely of non-complex carbohydrates and tend to promote an increase in our appetite. Complex carbohydrates help us to achieve a more even blood glucose level throughout the day. While "white foods" may be acceptable to some people who have no other options, these foods are a major source of calories in our diet and stimulate insulin and promote our hunger. They also tend to increase our blood sugar levels more dramatically. Foods made with whole grains have many proven advantages as already discussed.

Eliminating bread from your diet completely is another approach. I have become an advocate of the bread alternative, Crispbread, made with whole grain cereals. This is also referred to by some as Crackerbread. Often marketed as a product from Scandinavia, this low calorie food provides a more healthy mix of nutrients than one can easily obtain from regular bread. While there are many types of crispbread to choose from, one slice of crispbread made from 14 grams of whole grain rye flour contains 2 grams of fiber, 1 gram of protein, 0 grams of fat, 70 mg sodium, 11 grams of carbohydrate, and 45 calories. It also provides a healthy workout for your teeth and gums and promotes proper digestion and bowel function if eaten as a regular part of your diet instead of other forms of bread.

8. *Eliminate Fruit Juices From Your Diet and Substitute the Actual Fruit and Water*

Oranges and apples provide the necessary nutrients you are seeking yet without the added calories that accompany the fruit juice. It is amazing how few people appreciate the calories they are getting in their juice.

9. *Eat the Natural Product Itself*

If you prefer eating sweetened yogurt, fruit, or other foods, you can always add berries to provide a natural sweetener; beware manufacturers who add corn syrup, sugar of varying names and types, and other sweeteners that not only add calories but once again keep you craving for sweets in your diet. Break this cycle.

10. *Consider Innovative Alternate Choices*

If you crave ice cream, for example, my family has found a tasty lower calorie alternative that might appeal to you.

<u>Ice Cream Substitute</u>

Mix together:

Five ounces of fat-free evaporated milk

1/2 cup of frozen berries of your choice

1/2 banana, peeled, then frozen

Blend

This recipe makes 2 servings, each containing 62 calories, 0 grams fat, 0 grams cholesterol, 2 grams protein, and 4 grams carbohydrate

ENJOY!

Experiment and see what works for you as an alternative and healthier choice.

The *Be Fit for Life* Diet Plan

The following is a specially prepared diet option for those of you who want to try something different or have failed to achieve your goals after trying the suggestions listed above. This diet is intended for those of you who are aiming at a slow but steady loss of 2 to 3 pounds per week for a few months prior to switching to a maintenance diet plan that allows more choice of foods yet incorporates the principles of healthy eating and a well-balanced choice of nutrients as discussed throughout this book. All diet plans should be coupled with an exercise regimen that must be individually tailored to meet your unique abilities and goals.

The following diet plan has been carefully designed to emphasize foods that have been demonstrated to help achieve a more successful aging process and is called the "*Be Fit for Life Diet*". While this well balanced diet was designed to help promote weight loss, it can be used as a maintenance diet as long as you modify the calorie content to suit your needs. I hope that you will find this diet of great benefit and enjoy its variety of food options, colors, textures, and tastes, and choose to stay on it even after you have reached your weight goal. There is no harm, however, in using your new knowledge to branch out at this time and add variety to the suggested meals or substitute healthy choice alternatives. Use caution, however, to make sure you do not revert to your old eating habits.

The *Be Fit for Life Diet* contains a healthy and balanced source of calories and allows one to substitute for any meal a similar calorie choice. Some alternative options have been provided but you can make your own decisions using the knowledge you now have about healthy choices. Whey protein is suggested as a source of protein in several of the meals though alternate sources of protein, such as from soy, are also acceptable. Remember to practice Mindful Eating for maximal benefit! Prior to starting on this or any other diet, consideration should be given regarding pre-existing illness; this diet is not recommended for persons with pre-existing diseases of the kidney or liver.

The Be Fit for Life Diet should be part of a daily routine that includes a minimum of 30 minutes of exercise; drinking a sufficient quantity of water and/or club soda; and use of a supplemental daily multi-vitamin. It is comprised of 5 daily "meals" and depending on your individual goals can be modified as stated in the diet itself to provide anywhere between 1400 to 2500 calories daily. It will provide, unlike many other diets that are intended to "jump start" one's weight loss, beneficial quantities of protein, complex carbohydrates, fiber, vitamins and antioxidants. While this diet limits fat content to a healthy range, it does include the type and quantity of fat necessary to promote health and allow the body to metabolize calories maximally.

Meal 1

Taken as the first meal of the day, this meal should be complemented with a 30 minute exercise routine.

A. The first meal of the day is a shake consisting of 1 ounce (1 scoop) of whey or soy protein powder (depending on your preference), 3/4 cup raspberries (frozen) and 5 ounces of water with 3 ice cubes. All should be placed in a blender, mixed for 20 seconds, and enjoy! Providing 164 calories, this morning power shake provides the energy you need to "get going" and to stimulate your metabolism. It provides you with 22 grams of protein, 19 grams of carbohydrate, 0 grams of fat, and 4 grams of fiber.

B. Adding a medium sized banana to the above shake will add 110 calories while providing you with an additional 4 grams of fiber.

C. You should drink an additional 8 ounces of water at this time.

Individuals who wish to eat something with more consistency to start their day or who require a higher calorie content in their diet might consider additionally eating one or both of the following to complement the above shake:

D. Eat an apple. One medium sized, 2.5 inch, apple with the skin contains 80 calories, 5 grams of fiber, 21 grams of carbohydrate, 73 IU of vitamin A, 10 mg of calcium, 4 mg of Folic acid, and 8 mg of Vitamin C.

AND/OR

E. Eat one slice of crispbread topped with one slice, 28 grams, of low fat swiss cheese or its equivalent. This contains 95 calories, 2 grams fiber, 9 grams protein, 1 gram fat, 143 mg sodium, 2 grams fiber, and 12 grams carbohydrate.

Meal 2

This meal should be consumed mid-morning.

A. Oatmeal (1.62 ounces or 1/4 cup of Oat Groats, pre-cooked) plus ½ cup of hot/boiling water. One ounce (1 scoop) of whey protein powder or soy protein powder is sprinkled over the oatmeal and mixed in slowly. This provides 265 calories, 24 grams of protein, 4 grams of fiber and 0 grams of fat. If you have the ability to cook your oatmeal at this time of the day, I would suggest that you substitute a similar portion size of Steel Cut Oats for the pre-cooked Groats. Steel Cut Oats have a better metabolic effect on the body by being more slowly absorbed and less stimulating to endogenous insulin.

B. 8 ounces of unsweetened cranberry juice provides 60 calories and has a proven benefit on HDL levels. You can add 6 raspberries or blueberries to the oatmeal if you prefer and drink 8 ounces of water or club soda at this time.

C. Depending on the calorie requirements in your specific diet, a medium apple can be added to this meal. This provides 80 additional calories and 5 grams of fiber in the form of pectin.

Meal 3

This meal is best taken at lunch time and can vary somewhat depending on one's preferences and calorie requirements.

A. Yogurt (8 ounces, plain or vanilla/non-fat) is combined with 1/2 cup of raspberries, strawberries or blueberries (frozen or fresh). To this 1/3 cup of Oat Bran or Bran Buds is added.

B. One ounce or 2 tablespoons of almonds (approximately 6 almonds or equivalent as sliced or chopped almonds; 164 calories) can either be added to the Yogurt or taken afterwards recognizing the added calories that this provides.

This meal provides either 300 or 460 calories depending on whether you choose to add almonds and either 16.5 or 24.5 grams of protein, 6.5 or 19.5 grams of fiber, and 1 or 14 grams of fat.

C. Once again, drink 8 ounces of water or club soda with lemon at this time.

Meal 4

This meal is taken either late afternoon or as an early dinner.

A. A salad is made consisting of any amount you choose of the following: any form of lettuce, cucumber, snow peas, asparagus, cauliflower, green herb mixture, broccoli, or green beans. A "dressing" can be added consisting of vinegar, lemon juice and light, low-salt soy sauce if you choose to do so.

Any one of the following can be added to the salad. It is recommended that you vary your choice each day to provide more variety and balance. If you choose to use the broiling method of food preparation, use no more than one tablespoon of olive or canola oil in the pan and be sure to add spices to enhance the taste, such as garlic, basil, lemon grass, or sesame. Spray-on vegetable oils may help reduce the amount of oil necessary to keep the food from sticking to the cooking pan and are useful alternatives to the oil used in cooking.

Poached (see Poached Fish under Healthy Alternate Choices for Meal Substitution recipe), baked, broiled, or canned (3 oz in water) salmon; broiled or canned (3 oz in water) tuna; broiled or baked chicken breast without skin (3 oz); or tofu (3 oz).

B. A medium apple (80 calories) can be consumed either after the salad or cut up and sprinkled on top of the salad with the above options.

C. 8 ounces of unsweetened cranberry juice (60 calories), water, or club soda.

This meal, depending on your choice of salad "topping" provides between 225 and 360 calories, between 11.4 and 21.4 grams of protein, 1.5 and 5.1 grams of fat, and 11 grams of fiber.

For those who are seeking an even higher calorie content for their daily requirement, a larger portion of salmon, tuna, tofu or chicken may be used.

D. If one prefers or if calorie requirements mandate, a protein bar of one's choice may also be added to the diet at this time. This provides approximately 200 additional calories, 22 grams of protein, and 5 grams of fat, though will vary somewhat based on your choice of protein bar used.

Meal 5

Your day ends with another delicious protein shake. Best taken at least 2–3 hours prior to going to bed, this meal provides energy and muscle building components. If you were not able to exercise at the beginning of the day, this is the perfect time to do so!

A. One ounce (1scoop) of whey protein powder or soy protein powder is mixed with 2 tablespoons of almond or soynut butter and ½ cup of frozen raspberries, blueberries or strawberries. 5 ounces of water and 3 ice cubes are added prior to mixing for 45 seconds in a blender. This provides approximately 300 calories and 28 grams of protein, 16 grams of fat and 2 grams of fiber.

B. Drink an additional 8 ounces of water with lemon or unsweetened club soda at this time.

Those who require additional calories can add

C. Medium sized apple (approximately 80 calories)

AND/OR

D. Protein Bar (approximately 200 calories)

Additional comments:

While there is variation in this diet depending on one's daily choice of food from the suggestions made above, it can be individually tailored to provide between 1200 and 2,500 calories. These calories consist of a healthy proportion of protein (28–32%), carbohydrate (44–53%), and fat (21–24%), varying somewhat by the choices you have made from the options listed above. No saturated fats are included in this diet and depending on one's choice of foods and calorie requirements, it contains between 23 and 38 grams of fiber.

This diet should not only be considered by persons choosing to lose weight, however, as it provides a healthy and balanced nutritional plan. Even persons who choose to eat three meals a day rather than the 5 described above, can modify this diet to fit their desires and needs. For example, I find that the morning shake with a banana added provides me with energy and a full feeling that lasts until lunchtime. By slightly increasing the amount of what I eat at lunch and dinner and having only an apple as a mid-morning snack and an orange after dinner, I am able to maintain my desired number of calories and a content feeling throughout the day.

While the maximal amount of calories given for this diet plan is listed as 2,500 calories a day, individuals who want to remain on this diet though need a higher amount of calories can easily increase the portion size of any of the meals to add the desired number of calories or eat an additional protein bar, apple, choice of fruit, crispbread, or portion of yogurt to obtain their desired calories. The goal is to have you decide what is best for you based on the new knowledge you have learned about nutrition and making choices for a healthier YOU!

The following is a summary of how best to achieve the calories you strive for using the Be Fit for Life Diet Plan from the food selections listed above. Once again the calories listed are approximate and will vary somewhat based on your food preparation style and portion size used.

Meal	1,400 Calories Selections	1,600 Calories Selections	2,000 Calories Selections	2,500 Calories Selections
1	A and C	A, B, C, and D	A, B, C and D	A, B, C, D, and E
2	A and B	A and B	A, B, and C	A, B, and C
3	A and C	A and C	A, B, and C	A, B, and C
4	A and C	A and C	A, B, and C	A, B, C, and D
5	A and B	A and B	A, B, and C	A, B, C, and D

Healthy Alternate Choices for Meal Substitution

The following are just a few healthy alternative meal choices if you wish to substitute for any of the meals included in the *Be Fit for Life Diet* plan.

Yogurt and Oat Bran

An alternate choice for any of the above meals is 1/3 cup of oat bran mixed into 8 oz. of non-fat plain, vanilla, or strawberry yogurt. To add a special flavor, consider adding 1 tbs. of unsweetened jam or marmalade blended together though before doing so, consider that this "sweet" flavor may have consequences for those trying to break their "sweet habit" and is not an option for everyone. Stir contents until smooth. This provides a nourishing 180 calories, 15 grams of protein, 40 grams of carbohydrate, only 2 grams of fat and 4.5 grams of fiber.

One ounce of whey protein powder or soy protein powder can also be added for additional protein and calories. Adding one ounce of protein powder provides a meal with a total of 285 calories, 35 grams of protein, 45 grams of carbohydrate, 2 grams of fat and 4.5 grams of fiber.

Egg White Cheese Omelet on Oat Bran English Muffin

This is a delicious alternative to any of the meals listed above. It requires some cooking but is a healthy and filling substitute for an occasional meal.

Oat Bran English Muffins provide fiber and 5.0 grams of protein per muffin. Toast muffin and place on a plate.

Separate 3 egg whites from yolks and discard the yolks (a commercially available egg substitute can also be used). Stir until blended smoothly and pour into a hot pan sprayed lightly with vegetable cooking oil or that has a non-stick surface.

While heating, cut one slice of low-fat American or cheddar cheese (approximately 2/3 ounces) and place onto the egg surface. After one minute, fold sides of omelet over the cheese and then turn gently and heat a few minutes until done.

Serve on top of the English muffin and enjoy.

Provides 210 calories; 19.5 grams protein; 6.0 grams carbohydrate; 1.0 gram fat; and 2 grams fiber.

Poached Fish

This is one of my very favorite ways to prepare most types of fish and the recipe below was given to me by my wife who is a native Norwegian. Poached fish is rich in protein, omega oils, and naturally low in fat. Be careful how you prepare the fish and you are in for a delicious heart healthy and diet promoting meal. For many centuries, Scandinavians have enjoyed poaching their fish. Poached salmon has long been served at gourmet meals but you can enjoy this simple to make treat any day. Try using other firm, fleshy fish such as cod and haddock to make things interesting. Even mackerel and other more oily fish are delicious served in this manner, though they do require some additional seasoning.

Start with enough water just to cover the fish you will be poaching. Add approximately two teaspoons of salt and two tablespoons of lemon juice. Add 2–3 peppercorns, one bay leaf, 2–3 cloves of garlic and 2 pieces of clove. Bring the water to a boil and add 4 ounces of fish per serving- make sure that the heat is turned down after adding the fish and that the water is never allowed to boil again. Do not cover; simmer on low heat for approximately 15–20 minutes until done. Serve either warm or place in the refrigerator to cool for later use.

A 4 ounce portion of poached salmon provides approximately 200 calories; 27.6 grams protein; and 9.3 grams fat though only 70 mg cholesterol.

A 4 ounce portion of cod provides 119 calories; 25.9 grams protein; and only 1.0 gram fat of which 62 mg is cholesterol.

A 4 ounce portion of haddock contains 127 calories; 27.5 grams protein; and 1.1 gram fat of which 84 mg is cholesterol.

Note that I have listed a 4 ounce portion size above as compared to the 3 ounce portion of fish listed as an option for Meal 4 in the Be Fit for Life diet plan. Most individuals who are not on a "diet" consume at least 4 ounces of fish as a serving size with many choosing to increase this even more depending on preference and what else is being consumed in that meal. Remember to adjust the calories when adding up your totals based on your portion size. Fortunately, the difference in calories between 3 and 4 ounces of the above fish is minimal.

If you prefer mackerel or more "oily" fish, once again add a bay leaf, peppercorns, 2–3 cloves of garlic, 1 or 2 cloves and other favorings such as dill or basil depending on your taste preference as it simmers to bring out the flavor and reduce the "fatty" taste. Note that no oil has been added. A 4 ounce portion of mackerel cooked in this manner provides 300 calories; 27 grams protein; 20.2 grams fat of which 85 mg. is cholesterol.

Once you are done preparing the fish, it should be placed on a bed of any combination and portion size of any type of lettuce. You can add tomato and/or cucumber if you choose. During the summer months, take advantage of the wide variety of choices of lettuce; I also recommend using a green herb mixture as your base. While the "juices" of the poached fish may be sufficient, some will want to add a vinegrette prepared with vinegar, light soy sauce, and lemon.

Spinach and Garlic

Start with 9 ounces of baby spinach, washed, dried, and tough stems removed. Add finely chopped garlic (4 cloves). Sautee in a frying pan in 1 tablespoon of olive oil tossing gently until spinach is wilted. Depending on the surface of your cooking pan, more or less oil may be desirable. Serve. While this dish is rich in vitamins, minerals, and other nutrients, its caloric content is largely derived from the olive oil used in cooking. This recipe makes 2 servings each with approximately 110 calories; 3.0 grams protein; 4.5 grams carbohydrate; 4.0 grams fat; and 3.0 grams fiber. This dish is suggested as a complement to the dinner evening meal or as a healthy snack.

30

Next Steps for a More Successful Aging Process

Once you have committed yourself to change, taken stock in what you are currently doing, and decided where you need to go, you are already on the path to success. Whether or not your path will require you to lose weight, it is essential that you develop an exercise routine as well as consider the need to modify your existing lifestyle and diet. Your goals are within reach! The key, however, is to place yourself on a plan that will continue to suit your unique needs and one that you can stay on long term without any health consequences. If you do go on a weight reduction diet, you need to consider how best to transition at some point in time from a diet planned to help promote weight loss, whether it is the *Be Fit for Life Diet* or some other choice, to a diet that allows you a greater choice of foods and variety in food preparation. The principles listed above remain the same, however, and emphasize choosing foods that have proven health benefits, incorporate complex carbohydrates and fiber, liberal use of vegetables and fruits, controlled portion size, and restrict the use of fat, refined sugar, and other potentially unhealthy practices. These are diet tools that will help you to Be Fit for Life.

Many persons prefer to continue to keep the choice of their foods to a minimum thus reducing their chances of making a mistake. Others prefer to eat only pre-prepared foods that are bought with calorie and nutrition labels that clearly delineate what is included. Still others prefer to be in charge of their diet and are ready for the challenge. This is fine as long as the principles of dieting are adhered to and one is knowledgeable about what foods they will choose to eat as part of their lifelong diet plan.

As mentioned previously, most people needing to lose weight can readily classify themselves as being "Apples" or "Pears". Remember that "apples" tend to have more "central" obesity and heart disease; "pears" tend to have more diabetes due to a greater tendency to be insulin resistant. All forms of obesity pre-dispose one to hypertension. In fact, high blood pressure is a part of what is referred to as "Metabolic Syndrome". This disorder characterizes a person who has obesity, insulin resistance with or without diabetes, hyperlipidemia or high blood cholesterol, and hypertension. In all cases, a reduction in the absolute amount of calories to promote weight loss will be advantageous regardless of the composition of the diet. Weight loss will reverse the effects on these life-threatening factors; the longer someone is obese, the greater the chance of serious consequences.

Individuals who are "pears", accumulating buttock and thigh fat to a greater degree than fat in the abdomen, need to pay particular attention to their diet in order to avoid "refined sugars" and emphasize complex carbohydrates and foods with a lower glycemic index. Studies have shown a benefit of complex carbohydrates on insulin resistance, improving insulin sensitivity at the tissue level. Reducing the rapid swings of blood sugar that result from refined sugars is an advantage. Read labels carefully and avoid food products that contain corn syrup or are sweetened with "fruit juice", another term for fructose. Pay particular attention to the fat content in the diet and emphasize not only a reduction in total quantity but also try to use oils if required for cooking that have proven cardiovascular benefit such as canola or olive oil and in limited amounts. Do NOT eat fried foods and limit the amount of oil being used regardless of the form of cooking that is chosen. Restricting the sodium content in the diet will also be of benefit to many of those with co-existing hypertension or who tend to accumulate fluid; a "no added salt" regimen provides a good start for most.

For those who have been losing weight over the past few weeks and months and believe that they are ready to advance to the next step in their lifelong journey, a time when you can increase your choice of foods, choices must be made carefully based on health considerations, practical interests, with individual needs kept in mind. Clearly what will be allowed will depend on your calorie requirements. You must ask yourself if you are happy with the weight loss you have achieved to date and want to keep to the same number of calories you have been consuming or prefer to either increase or decrease the rate of weight loss you have been experiencing. Keep your expectations realistic and not overly ambitious; do not risk negative consequences to your health by eliminating key nutrients including sufficient calories necessary to promote a healthy immune system, muscle mass, and body function.

The decision is up to you. Remember, total calorie balance is the key to weight management and diet and exercise are the tools to achieve your goals! Choose wisely and seek assistance if you have questions or concerns. You are NOT alone!

If you have chosen to go on the *Be Fit for Life Diet* or some other diet and have achieved your desired goal of weight loss, consider making changes slowly as you increase your food choices and calories consumed. Perhaps each week substitute one of the meals that were part of the Diet Program with another well-balanced meal that emphasizes the principles listed above.

Try to incorporate as many foods as possible that have proven health benefits as listed in this book. While not always proven by well-conducted randomized controlled trials — the gold standard in scientific research — in most cases there is little to lose by choosing to include these foods.

Remember that circumstances may change during one's life and a diet plan that seemed "right" at one time may no longer be a viable or wise option. Whatever you choose, remember to be Mindful when eating and base your plan on your unique needs at the moment. You can always go back to some other diet plan when things change.

If you have followed my suggestions, you will find yourself eating more Mindfully, incorporating the practical suggestions I made for everyday eating, and are already eating a well-balanced diet built upon the principles referred to as a Mediterranean Diet and have included additional food choices with potential health benefit. This diet has stood the test of time and has been epidemiologically linked in large population studies to improved health and longevity. By being creative and finding ways to add healthy food items suggested in this book, you can continually improve upon your health and potential for a long and productive life.

As you embark on your lifetime of eating healthy, you may want to "fine-tune" your eating plan. Individuals who characterize themselves as overweight and "Pear" shaped, may want to emphasize more complex carbohydrates while restricting their total carbohydrate intake. Refined sugars should be avoided and there should be an emphasis on foods with soluble fiber, such as guar, oat bran, and pectin. There should also be an effort to reduce saturated fats in the diet and eat foods with a lower glycemic index.

Individuals who are overweight and describe themselves as "Apple" shaped should be most concerned about their cardiovascular health and would be well advised to lose weight, restrict saturated fats to no more than 10% of calories while limiting all fats to no more than 30%. Foods such as tofu, cranberries, cold water fish, soluble fiber, and oat bran should be encouraged to increase healthy cholesterol (HDL). Individuals with a strong risk of developing heart disease or those who already may have vascular illness may want to lower their fat intake ever further while also increasing their intake of soluble fiber and promoting weight loss to a desirable range. Adding limited amounts of dark chocolate, almonds, oranges, red grapes, de-caffeinated green tea, and a vegetable rich diet may also be useful tools to promote a more healthy heart.

Diet is not the only thing most people need to change in order to achieve a more successful aging process. Lifestyle modification, learning to cope with daily stressors, a daily exercise routine, getting a sufficient amount of restful sleep, and attention to aspects of your life that will help you avoid accelerating your otherwise "normal' aging process, prevent disease, and recognize and treat problems earlier are all necessary if we are to live happier, healthier, and more productive lives. While many ideas for achieving these goals have been delineated in this book, there are many other ways to accomplish these. The key is to have a goal in mind and understand why change may be necessary; the path to accomplishing your goals must remain an individual one and based on your own needs and specific abilities to accomplish them. Remember that YOU are in control of just how successful an aging process you will have. While you may not be able to change the genes you inherited from your parents and ancestors, each of us has the ability to maximize what we have been given.

The choice is up to YOU and the time to make a change is NOW!

About the Author
Steven R. Gambert, MD, AGSF, MACP

Dr. Gambert is a world recognized expert in the field of aging and geriatric medicine. He is a Professor of Medicine and Associate Chairman for Clinical Program Development in the Department of Medicine at the University of Maryland School of Medicine, where he is also Clinical Director of the Division of Gerontology and Geriatric Medicine and Director of Geriatric Medicine at the University of Maryland Medical Center and the world renowned R. Adams Cowley Shock Trauma Center. He is also Professor of Medicine, in the Division of Gerontology and Geriatric Medicine, Department of Medicine, at the Johns Hopkins University School of Medicine. A graduate of Columbia University College of Physicians & Surgeons in New York City, he did post-graduate training in Internal Medicine, gerontology/geriatric medicine, and endocrinology and metabolism at Dartmouth and Harvard Medical School affiliated programs.

Dr. Gambert has published extensively in the field of aging and has authored over 400 research articles, book chapters, and reviews. He is the Editor-in-Chief of Clinical Geriatrics, the clinical journal of the American Geriatrics Society. He has served in many leadership positions including being elected the President of the American Aging Association. He was elected a Master of the American College of Physicians, the most prestigious designation in Internal Medicine, and is a Fellow of the American Geriatrics Society and Gerontological Society of America. He has been consistently listed as one of the Best Physicians in America.

Dr. Gambert was one of the first investigators to study the endogenous opioid system and its relationship to aging, nutrition, exercise, and stress responses and is also well known for his original research relating to aging and the endocrine system. His research has additionally focused on improving our understanding of the aging process and medical care of the elderly. Dr. Gambert has additionally studied various aspects of Complementary and Alternative Medicine and in addition to being recognized and certified as an allopathic medical doctor (MD degree), he has been awarded the degree of Naturopathic Medical Doctor.

Index